14
cost

102
110
155

BOOK 5

ALL OUT AGAINST ARTHRITIS

ALL OUT
AGAINST
ARTHRITIS

by Faye C. Lewis, M.D.

PRENTICE-HALL, INC.
Englewood Cliffs,
New Jersey

All Out Against Arthritis by Faye C. Lewis, M.D.
Copyright © 1973 by Faye C. Lewis
Printed in the United States of America
Prentice-Hall International, Inc., London
Prentice-Hall of Australia, Pty. Ltd., North Sydney
Prentice-Hall of Canada, Ltd., Toronto
Prentice-Hall of India Private Ltd., New Delhi
Prentice-Hall of Japan, Inc., Tokyo

Library of Congress Cataloging in Publication Data

Lewis, Faye Cashatt.
  All out against arthritis.

  1. Arthritis. I. Title. [DNLM: 1. Arthritis—
Popular works. WE 344 L673a 1973]
RC933.L45   616.7'2   73–2683
ISBN 0–13–022392–1

10 9 8 7 6 5 4 3 2 1

Preface to the Reader

As you pick up this book from the bookstore table or library shelf and leaf through it, do not buy it with the expectation that it contains a magic cure for arthritis, hitherto unknown. I leave that to the charlatans. If such a thing existed, your own doctor would have told you.

Hopefully, however, I believe there are three benefits you may obtain from reading this book. First, it will give you a fuller understanding of the nature of arthritis—its history, symptoms, pathology, and its supposed possible causes, which are still a matter of controversy.

Second, it should give you some reassurance that you are not suffering from a malady so common that no one pays any attention to it. That day is thankfully past—a part of the dark ages of arthritis. This is a new day, with new hope and promise, implemented by as much determination and concentrated effort as have ever been brought to bear against any disease. Previous successes in campaigns for the eradication of other diseases should inspire confidence in this one.

Third, whatever the type and severity of your arthritis, this book should leave no doubt in your mind that there are things that can be done for you. And there are even more important things that you can do for yourself.

—FAYE C. LEWIS, M.D.

Acknowledgments

The following publications furnished source material for this book: *Modern Trends in Rheumatology; Medical World News; The Woman Physician; Chronic Disease Management; Journal of the American Medical Association; Chemical and Engineering News; New England Journal of Medicine; Medical Insight; Journal of Chronic Diseases; Adult and Child; Tri-state Medical Journal; Proceedings of the Institute of Medicine, Chicago; British Medical Journal; Arthritis and Rheumatism; Archives of Internal Medicine; Archives of Family Practice.*

Evelyn Duro prepared the manuscript for submission to the publisher. Marion Samo, of the Iowa State Medical Library, found much interesting material on the history of arthritis and made copies for me. Michael New, Field Director of the Iowa Chapter of the Arthritis Foundation, supplied me with the concise and authoritative manuals compiled by that organization. Mrs. Mary Hanna and her staff of the Kendall Young Library gave me capable assistance upon many occasions.

Contents

To Diane, my encouragement factor

Part One

ARTHRITIS—Background and Definitions

I

The History of Arthritis

My previous experience and knowledge of arthritis had been that of a practicing physician: seeing patients with all degrees of involvement and suffering, searching hopefully through the current medical literature for clues to a better understanding of the problems and more efficient treatment approaches, attending an occasional seminar for advice and opinions from leading authorities on the subject.

All my attention had been centered upon human beings, of course. I knew in a vague way that domestic animals had arthritis, too, from chance remarks of friends and patients about their ailing pets. I knew, also, that arthritis is one of the most dreaded diseases of racehorses. (I had even made that snap diagnosis on several horses I had bet on at Florida Downs.)

When the scope of my reading widened, I learned that arthritis has left the most ancient pathological records in existence for any disease. Along with this knowledge came the realization that from the point of time, *human* arthritis occupies only an infinitesimal part of the history of arthritis in general. Human arthritis is one of the newer things under the sun, just as human beings themselves are upstarts among the living creatures that have occupied the earth.

The most ancient examples of arthritis occur in the early reptilian vertebrates of a hundred million years ago, whose spinal columns show the fusings and erosions of the diseased vertebrae much as they occur today. These findings appear to support the gloomy conclusion that aching backs have existed about as long as the spinal columns themselves. If these creatures could have known what awaited their ambitious descendants, one wonders whether they might not have melted back amorphously into the ooze.

The oldest known evidence of multiple arthritis also dates back about a hundred million years (give or take a few million, as the scientists say guardedly). It is a prized specimen in a basement room of the Museum of Natural History on the campus of the State University in Lawrence, Kansas.

I had read many more details about this specimen than I would have been able to observe at a distance of a foot or two, through a glass case; details both macroscopic and microscopic, recorded by trained observers in the field. But I had never quite convinced myself. Nevertheless, having done all available reading, seeing seemed the final knowledge that would nail a trophy immutably to the walls of memory.

Circumstances aligned themselves in my favor. Driving home from Florida in the first week in March, we ran into a snowstorm in Kansas City. Visibility was

4

so poor that we stopped early for the night. The next morning was sunny; the fog lifted, and our spirits with it, and it seemed no arduous task at all to detour the short distance to Lawrence before continuing on home.

So here we stood, my husband and I, before a long glass case, gazing at this gouty platycarpus, member of the family of mosasaurs. (I have no authority for my diagnosis of gout, since none of the recorded findings attempt to classify the type of arthritis. It is the location of the pathology, in the joints of the toes, that has led me to think of it this way.)

One feels a certain awe in looking at something a hundred million years old. It boggles the mind to try to stretch that far back. This skeleton we were looking at was naked antiquity.

"I hadn't expected it to be so large," I said, after a moment. "It must be fifteen feet long."

"More like twenty feet," my husband replied, and stepped off the distance, verifying the accuracy of his estimate.

The skeleton is complete, no bones missing; the skull with its long ferocious-looking jaws, the rudimentary limbs, the row of vertebrae extending with a graceful diminuendo in size to the tip of the tail. The bones are set in a matrix, and the entire exhibit tilted at about half a right angle, to facilitate viewing by visitors. The completeness of the skeleton seems sufficient proof that it must have lain for these million centuries undisturbed by the disruptive changes occurring on the earth surface above it, including the more gentle stirrings of the topsoil in the cultivation of Kansas wheat.

A few paleontologists have specialized in the diseases that occurred among the early fossil animals they have unearthed. Notable among these was Dr. Roy Lee

Moodie, whose writings include two textbooks on paleopathology. It is from these few paleontologists who paid special attention to the evidences of disease in their specimens that we have learned what we know about the oldest examples of arthritis in existence. Arthritis, of course, lends itself peculiarly well to study after long periods of time, since it involves the bones, which do not disintegrate as do the soft parts of a specimen. Therefore, although the vast amount of extant evidence seems to indicate that arthritis has been a very common disease throughout the ages, there is nothing to show how its incidence compared with that of other diseases of those times (such as cancer, tuberculosis, or virus infection) which, involving only the soft parts, may have afflicted or even killed their hosts without leaving a trace of their identity.

The mosasaurs have left no descendants; they are completely extinct. What happened to them is a matter of speculation, with no proof. Some cataclysmic geophysical occurrence is a handy assumption, but some paleopathologists have wondered whether the high incidence of arthritis might not have been a factor. It seems an idea worthy of consideration. The pain, swelling, and stiffness in the mosasaurs' joints must surely have impeded their search for food, as well as their swimming away from their enemies.

The evidence of the existence of arthritis in these early vertebrates makes quite an impact on our concept of the times they lived in. Writing in the *Archives of Internal Medicine,* Drs. Robert S. Karsh and J. D. McCarthy philosophize gloomily that our mental picture of a happier age, when carefree creatures roamed the pristine earth in blissful ignorance of troubles, aches, and pains to come, must be a false one. It is

6

unlikely that such an idyllic epoch ever existed. A far truer picture, they say, can be painted "of grotesque reptilian monstrosities limping, not cavorting, through the jungles and swamps to bathe their sick joints in the warm muck of the natural spas that surrounded them." Thus my visit to the museum gave me what I had hoped for, a visual contact with the beginnings of this invidious disease that has tortured the vertebrate forms of life since their start on earth.

While there I met a man who had known Dr. Roy Lee Moodie well; had, in fact, been a pupil of his. This was Dr. Edward H. Taylor, herpetologist at the museum. Among his personal reminiscences, he told me that Dr. Moodie himself had suffered severely from arthritis, and that it was in Dr. Moodie's classes in zoology that he had felt the impetus that directed him into his own career. These two statements, it seems to me, epitomize the finest type of scientist: a man who can retaliate constructively against his own miseries by spending his lifetime mining information to add to the stockpile of weaponry being assembled toward the annihilation of the disease, and at the same time inspiring his students to accomplishments beyond his own.

Ambition must have been one of the strongest stimuli operative in the evolution of man, stirring one group of primates to learn to ambulate on their two hind legs, reserving their front extremities for more specialized uses. And how these uses multiplied: from the innocence of nurturing and toolmaking to the evils of aggression and weaponry, and reaching their height in the arts.

These ambitions, too, have had their punishments. Standing proudly on the two hind legs imposed the total body weight on the knees, and maintaining this erect posture involved some curvings of the spine. If these early primates could have foreseen that these two adaptations were inviting the agonies of arthritis, might they not have been content to continue getting about on all fours? The answer, of course, is no. Ambition knows no reins. It forges ahead against all hazards, even to technological marvels capable of destroying the race.

Almost everything else in nature undergoes evolutionary changes, but not arthritis. The disease that affected the reptiles of a hundred million years ago shows the same distortions and erosions in the joints it attacks as in prehistoric man.

The earliest evidence of arthritis in any biological specimen that could be called human goes back to the Java man, unearthed by Eugene Dubois in the late 1800's. The Java man's age is estimated at no more than a half-million years. His pathology consists of outgrowths of bone at the upper end of the left thighbone, at the site of muscle attachments. There is no evidence of joint erosions. These findings have given rise to the opinion that this earliest known human arthritic probably did not suffer much from his affliction.

The first truly human sufferer from arthritis was the Neanderthal man, the original *Homo sapiens.* Nor is there any question as to the suffering in his case. An examination of one Neanderthal skeleton leaves no doubt. He had a fracture at the upper end of the larger bone in his left forearm, which healed, but left a stiff and misshapen elbow joint. One hopes, sympathetically, that he was right-handed! These Neanderthal specimens show the degenerative type of arthritis, which nearly a century ago came to be labeled osteoarthritis. It has been present in man ever since his existence, demonstrable in almost any of the exhumed civilizations—Egyptian, Peruvian, pre-Columbian Indian—wherever astute observers with an eye for pathology take the trouble to look for it.

The most ancient acceptable pathological specimen of rheumatoid arthritis was unearthed in Egypt by Professor Flinders Petrie and reported in the *British Medical Journal* in 1897. The source of these findings was a carefully wrapped mummy, a man who had died at about fifty years of age, who had been lying in the middle of a Deshasheh cemetery, interred amid ceremonial statues of Nen Kheft Ka, to propitiate the gods, where he lay undisturbed for forty-seven hundred years. The hands that disinterred him, however, were probably none the less reverent for being inspired by science instead of religion.

Two of history's oldest arthritics identified by name were the Egyptian Nefermaat, and Ashurbanipal, an Assyrian. Nefermaat had the ankylosing or fixation type of arthritis, his entire spine being solid and inflexible from the neck down. In Egyptian hieroglyphic writing, the symbol used to denote old age was the picture of a man deformed from chronic arthritis. One of the earliest medical recommendations on record is a clay tablet found in the palace of Ashurbanipal, suggesting a fomentation of rotten and fermenting barley to be sat in for relief of arthritic back pain.

Arthritis must have been taken for granted by the ancients, considered a part of the process of aging. It is doubtful that it was thought to be a separate disease, for no one troubled to record any history or commentary on it until the time of Hippocrates. To him, one of the most noteworthy characteristics of arthritis was the predilection it had for the aged.

But the questioning mind of Hippocrates, "Father

of Medicine," did some probing into the possible causes of this affliction, and he attributed arthritis in the Scythians to trauma to the joints resulting from excessive horseback riding. After these observations of Hippocrates, it seems incredible that a thousand years were to elapse before there was any continued persistent study of the disease, only the sporadic, happenstance notations of a number of scientists. As Jean Martin Charcot said: "Disease is very old, and nothing about it has changed. It is we who change as we learn to recognize what was formerly imperceptible."

The Emperor Diocletian once issued an edict that citizens severely afflicted by arthritis need not pay taxes! One wonders about his motives. Was he the sympathetic and humane man that this would make him appear? We must recall Diocletian's cruelty to women and children when necessary to achieve an end, his persecution of the Christians, and his final voluntary relinquishment of power for the serene enjoyment of raising cabbages in his garden. Or was Diocletian himself a sufferer from arthritis, and thus making provision for a possible future need of his own? Besides attempting to relieve the financial burdens of arthritics, he absolved citizens crippled with gout from strenuous physical duties.

Quintus Ennius, a poet born of Greek and Italian parentage, was brought to Rome in his youth by Cato, to write voluminously in many poetic forms. His epic history of Rome became the national poem of Italy until the time of Virgil. Ennius was severely afflicted with arthritis, and died of gout at the age of seventy. One wonders what kind of poetic inspiration would be felt by a man undergoing such suffering, and whether his writing might not reflect some bitterness and resentment. One irreligious statement of his might be an expression of such feeling: "I grant you there are gods, but they don't care what men do; else it would go well with the good and ill with the bad, which rarely happens." He composed this proud epitaph for himself:

Pay me no tears, nor for my passing grieve;
I linger on the lips of men, and live.

The most famous quotation from the works of Ennius is, "Never a poet unless arthritic." He was the first to make this philosophical adaptation to his miseries, giving many who came after him a rule to live by: "If you can't rid yourself of your affliction, then wear it like a badge of honor."

Some notable arthritics have come down in history. One of these was Piero de Medici, who was called Piero the Gouty. He was reported to have been so severely afflicted that old records say of him, "His tongue alone retained any motion." Like Ptolemy Philadelphus, he passed this unfortunate predilection for joint trouble along to a great many of his descendants. Lorenzo the Magnificent forfeited his claim to magnificence while still young in years and became a decrepit, crippled old man. Fate dealt similarly with the meteoric, Catherine de Medici, who became toothless and arthritic in her decline.

Cardinal Richelieu's amazing history takes on a gloomy note as one reads details of his personal health. He is said to have been one of the most constipated men on record, and suffered throughout his life from hemorrhoids, a common accompaniment of chronic constipation. Topping these miseries, he had a shifting arthritis, which settled in his jaw joints. Reading such histories as these, one wonders whether greatness is

11

nurtured more often by ease and comfort, or by the proddings of suffering.

Some of the world's most famous soldiers were arthritic, among them Julius Caesar, Alexander Farnese, Frederick the Great. Thus the same adjustment should be made in our thinking about these military stalwarts as about the arthritic prehistoric monsters. As they swaggered on parade it was sometimes to the accompaniment of painful, creaking joints, not always the display of unflawed physical fitness that they appeared to be.

The list of notable arthritics could go on and on, with the addition of such names as the Prince of Condé, François de La Rochefoucauld, Benvenuto Cellini, William Pitt, John Calvin, and Peter Paul Rubens. The thought occurs to the researcher that the number might be multiplied if as meticulous records had been kept of the ailments of these famous people as of their accomplishments, and that probably we know only of the most severely afflicted, not of the comparatively minor cases. It is small wonder that the ancients felt that a man could not be truly great unless arthritic, that, in effect, arthritis was the painful initiation fee exacted from those selected to the Society of the Great.

Although there was no generalized study of arthritis between the time of Hippocrates and the beginning of the nineteenth century, some progress was made, however halting it was. Looking back upon these sparse findings, it is evident that a pattern of differentiation was beginning to emerge which eventually was to relegate the word "rheumatism" to the scientific scrap heap as being too general for practical use. To some extent it survives in the parlance of the general public, where it means anything that causes distress in the arms, legs, or back, which might be any one of a hundred or more pathological conditions. Nonetheless, each of a number of observers contributed his specific bit to make an aggregate of some value. Among this group, the name of Thomas Sydenham looms large in importance. He recorded the first *clinical* description of rheumatoid arthritis.

David Douglas, for whom the Douglas fir is named, made a unique contribution to the annals of arthritis. He was a nineteenth-century botanist whose love of adventure coupled with his botanical explorations was the dominant impulse in his life. He discovered gold in California seventeen years before the gold rush began, but was quite unconcerned by it, giving little thought to the flecks of yellow metal clinging to the roots of one of the California pines he was packing for shipment. He kept a journal throughout his extensive travels by ship, horseback, canoe, and on foot. He was twenty-five years old when he began having arthritis in his knees. From then on, for the next ten years, his journals are dotted with reports of painful involvement in various joints, sometimes to the point where he was incapacitated for a time, together with a record of the physical rigors attendant upon his travels—cold, fatigue, lack of shelter, minor accidents—an account which is painful even to the reader but at the same time a valuable blow-by-blow story of rheumatoid arthritis. He became despondent at times, although not to the point of giving up his work. On New Year's Day, 1826, he wrote, "In all probability, if a change does not take place, I will shortly be consigned to the tomb." He was then twenty-seven years old. He met a violent end at the age of thirty-six, presumably gored to death by a wild bull.

There are no boundaries to the effects of arthritis

13

today. They extend far outside the home, permeating our entire society—our schools, hospitals, rehabilitation centers, charitable institutions, churches, industry, employment agencies, insurance companies, businesses of all sort. Any disease that does not kill its victims, but almost insures them a long, handicapped life, is beyond the capacity of most families to handle by themselves. The responsibilities, especially the financial ones, must spill over into society.

The extent of this social burden is almost beyond our mental grasp. The Arthritis Foundation has furnished us with some breathtaking figures about this number-one crippling disease in our nation. At any one time, there are about a million and a half people disabled by arthritis; over twelve million days lost from work annually; a quarter of a million new victims each year. The annual cost of arthritis to the national economy approaches four billion dollars.

2

Nature of the Affliction

An attempt to actually *define* arthritis as a disease-entity becomes an exercise in frustration. We thought we were taking a scientific step forward when we discarded the old term "rheumatism," which referred vaguely to the overflowing of painful "humors" into the tissue, which caused aching. We were much happier with the term "arthritis," which means joint inflammation. We thought that at least we had the pathology nailed down. But the more we learn about arthritis, the more we add to the confusion of terminology. As an amateur botanist might place in one category all the plants that bear red berries, then learn upon more advanced study that, in fact, they represent many different plant families, so the physician researcher finds that arthritis is the baleful fruit of a great number of diseases, sometimes estimated as high as a hundred.

The starting point out of this maze is an understanding of the bones and joints themselves—their structure, functions, and the ways in which they differ from the other parts of the body. One outstanding characteristic of the bone-joint system is that its role in the body is a passive one. Preposterous as it may sound at first, the bones and joints do nothing active. Their job is to support the body structure, to hold things up, to hang things on, to fasten things to. The bones have no power of motion within themselves; it is the muscles that do the work. One of the tiresome disciplines facing the young anatomy student is learning by rote the names of the muscles attached to each bone, and the exact location of each attachment. Parts of the skeletal system afford protection to the vital organs. The rib cage shields the heart and lungs against external injury. The spinal column is analogous to the concrete tunnel for the safe conduct of the body's communication system, while the skull is the safety vault for the brain. In a sense, a motorcyclist's helmet gives him an accessory skull.

The skeletal system's own defense against harm is largely a built-in one—its density of structure allows it to absorb many a hard knock. But while this hard compactness is effective against *external* injury, it makes the skeletal system vulnerable to attacks from within. The other, so-called "soft parts" of the body depend largely upon their rich nerve and blood supply, for protection as well as for nourishment. In case of any kind of threat, messages can be sent telling accurately the location of the danger, insuring prompt action to the rescue. If the enemy is a bacterial invasion, there is an immediate multiplication of white blood cells, seemingly out of nowhere, massed for attack against the invaders. If the trouble is traumatic—a cut or bruise—

the injured area is walled off and new tissue begins to form.

The skeletal system is much less richly supplied with nerves and blood vessels. Our usual assumption is that bones and joints are tough, that all they need is sufficient nourishment and they can get along on their own—which, for the most part, they can. But being left to "rough it" without any more than the minimum attentive care of the nerves and blood vessels, it takes them longer to recover when damage does occur; their devastation lasts longer. A broken bone, for example, takes much longer to heal than a cut muscle.

The skeletal system of the body is composed of an assortment of two hundred and some bones, articulated together with exquisite precision. Some of these joinings are fixed, as in the bones of the skull. Many of the others are much more complicated in structure, to meet the requirements for free and intricate mobility. When we speak of the joints, of their stresses, their diseases and their problems in general, it is almost always these movable joints that we have in mind.

The first requisite for an efficient movable joint is that the ends to be articulated must be contoured to fit snugly together. Covering the surface of these contoured ends is a layer of rubbery gristle, called cartilage. This cartilage layer varies in extent with the stage of development of the bone. In young growing bones, it acts as a matrix for the bone formation, gradually becoming impregnated with calcium, and hardens, thus increasing the size of the bone. In bones that have achieved their full growth, the role of the cartilage layer is limited to its cushioning action in the joint.

Whenever two parts of the body are in frequent contact, there must be an emollient—or lubricating—

protection. The eyeballs are bathed in secretions from the tear ducts to keep the constant motion of the lids from being abrasive. The mouth is kept moistened by the salivary glands. The vaginal canal is surfaced with mucus (a wise provision of nature sometimes defeated by women who have a fetish for cleanliness). The joints, in turn, are kept "oiled" by synovial fluid encapsulated about them. The surface of the cartilage layer is smooth, and the synovial fluid bathing it makes it slippery.

The ends of the bones are held in apposition at the joint by strands and bands of tough, dense fibers called ligaments, and the entire joint is boxed into a capsule of this same ligamentary tissue and lined by a softer membrane which secretes the synovial fluid.

Given these requisites for a normal, smoothly moving joint, let us consider what may happen to impair its function.

The joints take the brunt of most of the stresses on the skeletal system, and they often suffer from the prolonged weight-bearing and friction. (An obese patient with arthritis of the knees is always advised to lose weight as part of this treatment.) Cartilage changes are usually first to occur. After long use, the cartilage may become frayed or pitted in spots. It loses its resilience, becomes less springy, and this, in turn, makes it less able to cope with weight and motion. Instead of flexing with these stresses, it remains inert under them, becomes more and more vulnerable to their eroding effects. These wear it thinner and thinner, and in some places leave bare spots in the bone ends, completely denuded of the protective cartilage.

The function of the joint is now in serious jeopardy. Having lost the smoothness of the gliding surfaces, movement of the joint becomes painful. Protective mechanisms now go into action—which, in this instance, make matters worse. One of the gambits the body employs to shield a distressed area is a buildup of fortifying tissue.

The most easily demonstrated results of this action are on the skin. Hard-working hands acquire a protective horniness. Friction from ill-fitting shoes causes corns and calluses—not pleasant themselves, but better than having areas of skin worn off. A similar stir of recuperative action can take place about a damaged joint. Being unable to grow smooth new patches over the worn areas of cartilage, the body does the best it can, thickening bony tissue over the denuded bone ends, sometimes in spurs of new bone where the ligaments and capsule are attached.

This stop-gap activity changes the contours of the joint surfaces, impairing the mobility of the joint sometimes to the point of making it completely dysfunctional. But further damaging complications may occur. Cysts may form in the ends of the bones near the joint, causing other distortions in shape, and thinning some surface areas of bone. Bits of bone and cartilage may break off and fall loose into the joint cavity. Any of these possibilities means further deterioration in the usefulness of the joint.

All the indications of trouble in a joint are technically labeled "arthritis," although the meaning of the word is limited to *inflammation*. The classical signs of inflammation are heat, redness, swelling, and pain. These symptoms occur with enough regularity both singly and in groups, in joint disease to justify the conclusion that what we commonly call arthritis is indeed a matter of inflammation in most if not all cases. The exceptions, however, (even if few in number), are enough to make us look carefully, lest important factors be ignored.

Pain may be the patient's first awareness that there is something wrong with a joint, but it is not the first thing that has happened. Obviously, something must have occurred to cause the pain. The discomfort may be only recurrent twinges, a dull ache, or a constant suffering severe enough to immobilize the joint. The site of the most severe pain may not be in the joint itself but in adjacent muscle groups. Arthritis of the shoulder, for example, may cause an ache most noticeable in the muscles of the upper arm.

The afflicted joints often swell, sometimes to the extent that fluid may be withdrawn with a syringe. The joints themselves may be red and hot to the touch, although this latter finding is not one of the most common ones. There is usually some stiffness, and some limitation of motion.

When joint trouble reaches the chronic stage, a grating may be felt under the examiner's hand as the affected joint is moved. Sometimes motion is accompanied by an audible creaking. However, this seldom attains the noise level as in one patient of mine who had been partially immobilized for several years from arthritis in most of her joints. When she told me how much her joints creaked, I thought she must be exaggerating—until she demonstrated for me. When her left shoulder was moved passively by the nurse, I could hear the creak plainly from the room across the hall!

With the advance of the trouble, the affected joints may become stiffer and stiffer to the point of being fixed and immovable, with horrible accompanying distortions. Many early arthritics are haunted by the image of some pitiable patient they have known, lying gnarled and helpless in bed, with little motility left in any part of the body. To be told that these severe cases are greatly in the minority affords only some degree of reassurance.

A patient with any combination of the joint signs mentioned here seldom comes to the physician asking, "What is wrong with me, doctor?" Arthritis is one of the few afflictions that brings the patient in with a statement instead of a question. As he can put a name to it himself, why ask the doctor? His approach is more apt to be, "I think I've got a touch of arthritis," or "My arthritis is flaring up again"—in which the physician concurs. What the patient wants is "something to take for it."

This, in general, is the train of events that occurs in osteoarthritis. Any of the joints may be affected, but the ones most commonly involved are those that bear weight, such as the knees, hips, and spine. It frequently occurs also in the joints at the base of the thumb and big toe, and in the terminal joints of the fingers. Bony bumps, called Heberden's nodes, may appear at these terminal finger joints, making the diagnosis of osteoarthritis evident at a glance. These nodes are usually painless, but one osteoarthritic joint in the hand that may be quite uncomfortable is the one at the base of the thumb. The pain may be exacerbated by any tensing, gripping motion of the hand, such as wringing out a washcloth. I had one patient whose chief complaint was the pain at the base of her right thumb, starting each summer in the sweet corn season. The firmness of the grip of her thumb and the first two fingers, necessary to pull the husks off the ears, was sufficiently irritating to that joint to cause constant pain. She was a stubborn

Norwegian, however, and never stopped serving sweet corn to her family during the season.

There may be more than one basis for the classification of a disease. Thus, while osteoarthritis obviously belongs with the other joint diseases, there would be some justification for linking it with arteriosclerosis, or "hardening of the arteries" commonly observed in the old. The wear and tear of long continued use is the chief causative factor of each. They are diseases of the aging, and we all get them if we live long enough.

In arteriosclerosis, increasing amounts of connective tissue become knitted into the walls of the blood vessels, making them firmer and less elastic. The pathology of osteoarthritis is of a different nature entirely, reflecting the different make-up of the joints themselves and the effects of the particular stresses to which they are subject.

One good thing about osteoarthritis as opposed to the other arthritic diseases is that it is always localized. It does not cause systemic symptoms of illness, as many of the others do. But in a sense, it seems logical to place upon it some of the blame for our retarded knowledge of many of these other diseases. Osteoarthritis is so widespread that for centuries it has been confused with a number of rarer types, capable of much more damage to the human body in general. Slowly and painfully our scientific explorers have been ferreting these out, subjecting them to individual scrutiny as to characteristics and possible causes. Each newly identified member of this pernicious family gives more weight to the possibility that a new classification system may be in the offing.

With a new case of arthritis in his office, the physician must first categorize it as to type. To which of the known families of arthritis does it belong? Following the leads suggested by the case history, the state of health of many other parts of the body must be probed —including such widely separated areas as the kidneys, heart, even the eyes—before the question can be answered satisfactorily. In other words, the type of arthritis dictates the treatment and directs the attention to parts of the body that may be involved, in addition to the joints.

But even proper identification of the family group to which the case belongs falls far short of giving a clear picture of its backgrounds. There are murky areas in all these groups, each a wilderness of unanswered questions with its jungle underbrush of false concepts, misleading trails, and even superstition. Steady progress is being made, however. The wilderness is being mapped, pertinent signs noted, and guideposts set up for future use, to which each carefully studied case contributes its quota, statistically if not in the area of new discovery.

Part Two

*Types of Arthritis and
How They Behave*

3

Gout

Numerous treatises on arthritis have been written by physicians suffering from it, writing from bitter personal experience. Most notable among these was Thomas Sydenham, who has been called "The English Hippocrates." He suffered throughout most of his adult life from gout, and is thought to have died from kidney complications of it. His writing shows that vividness of description possible only to the physician who has observed the symptoms in himself. He speaks of pain "like the gnawing of a dog," which may have been the inspiration for an advertisement for gout medication in a recent medical journal. It shows a grisly picture of a distorted, swollen foot being gnawed upon by rats.

The mental picture that gout suggests to almost everyone is that of a greatly swollen big toe—a picture in which there is quite a bit of scientific accuracy. Although gout may attack any of the joints, those of the hands and feet, especially those of the big toe, are most commonly affected. One logical explanation given for the predilection of gout for this site is that an especially high pressure per square inch is exerted on the joint at the base of the big toe in walking—another example of the deleterious effects of stress.

The word "gout" comes from the Latin *gutta,* meaning a drop. According to the old humoral theory of the disease, the swelling increased drop by drop, hence the name. But the "drop by drop" description suggests too gradual an onset, and must have come from an observer, not from one of the sufferers. Patients reporting on their own illness often mention being suddenly jolted awake by pain in the middle of the night.

This is how Thomas Sydenham described it. His treatise on gout is one of the classics of seventeenth-century medicine:

> The victim goes to bed and sleeps in good health. About two o'clock in the morning he is awakened by a severe pain in the great toe; more rarely in the heel, ankle or instep. The pain is like that of a dislocation, and yet the parts feel as if cold water were poured over them. Then follow chills and shivers, and a little fever. The pain, which was at first moderate, becomes more intense. With its intensity, the chills and shivers increase. . . . Now it is a violent stretching and tearing of the ligaments—now it is a gnawing pain and now a pressure and a tightening. So exquisite and lively meanwhile is the feeling of the part affected, that it cannot bear the weight of the bedclothes nor the jar of a person walking in the room.

This excruciating pain, accompanied by joint swelling, was enough to set gout apart as the earliest specialized form of arthritis to be recognized, in fact one of the earliest diseases of any kind to be recognized by man. It was described in writings thousands of years ago. Rheumatologists, as researchers in the arthritic diseases are sometimes called, have reason to be proud of their record in gout, since this is the first of this group of diseases to be brought under control. It has not been wiped out, and is not even curable in the permanent sense; but attacks can now be aborted and even warded off for long periods.

Gout presents definite and easily detectable systemic signs, demonstrated in the laboratory. For some reason, as yet unknown, the body chemistry goes awry in one respect, resulting in too high a concentration of uric acid in the body fluids. The manufacture of uric acid in the body is a normal life process, and hence uric acid is a normal constituent of the body; but in gout either too much is produced, and/or the excess is not thrown off efficiently by the kidneys. Uric acid is not readily soluble in body fluids, and in higher than normal concentrations it will separate out in the form of tiny crystals of sodium urate, a uric acid salt. These crystals collect in the joints and also in the kidneys. In addition to the pain and swelling they cause in the joints, they can cause damage to kidney tissue and contribute to the formation of kidney stones. The picture of a collection of these relatively hard crystals gritting about in the soft body tissues is a horrendous one, sufficiently convincing of their capabilities for pain and destruction.

One of the simplest tests for the presence of too

much uric acid in the blood was devised by A. B. Garrod in 1847. He immersed a string in a gouty patient's blood serum, and collected uric acid crystals on it.

In some chronic cases of gout, another derivative of uric acid, a white, chalky substance, may be deposited in the tissues, usually in or about the joints (especially the elbow), or at the rims of the ears. They are usually painless, and the ones in the rims of the ears feel to the palpating finger like BB shot buried under the skin. These are called *tophi,* and the pathological condition in which they occur is known as tophaceous gout. One woman who had tophaceous deposits protruding from the knuckles of her hand was able to write on a blackboard with her closed fist!

Uric acid is made out of substances called purines, some of which are manufactured in the body, and some of which are present in foods. As is logically to be expected in view of these findings, diet plays a role in the control of gout. This has always been suspected, however, even before anything was known about purines or uric acid. In earliest times, gout was supposed to be a hazard of rich living. This theory has now been moderated, as have all our ideas as to the significance of diet in this disease. Whatever role diet plays, it is now the universal opinion that it is secondary to that of drugs. To be on the cautious side, the kind of meal a gouty patient should avoid is one with liberal helpings of sweetbreads, brains, kidney, or liver, washed down with large quantities of beer—all these edibles being high in purines. The dietary restrictions on which most doctors would agree are the avoidance of alcoholic binges, which have appeared to provoke acute attacks, and overeating. On the other hand, it would not be possible to eliminate from the diet all the substances from which the body can manufacture uric acid; and sudden, painful attacks have been known to occur during the strictest possible abstention from purines. Obesity is an unfavorable condition in the control of gout, as well as most other diseases; in fact, obesity is an unfavorable body condition in general.

Gout is an inheritable disease in the same sense that many other diseases are "inherited." Whatever body weakness fosters the overproduction of uric acid and/or the kidneys' inability to throw off the excessive amounts of it may be passed along from one generation to the next. Not everybody with high uric acid levels in his blood, gets gout, however. So there must be other factors involved, one or more of those unknowns that infest the entire field of arthritic diseases.

The existence of unknowns in any branch of medicine is always a continuing reproach, and at the same time a prodding to the discovery of their identity. In 1666, Daniel Sennert called gout "opprobrium medicorum," the physician's shame—because it was so infrequently recognized. Another name for gout, "podagra," was descriptive in quite a different sense. Its derivation was meant to convey the idea "caught in a trap."

Gout is a man's disease. No more than five percent of the cases occur in women. Women have lower average uric acid levels than men, which is significant but not particularly revelatory in a causative sense.

One theory that has enjoyed some popularity is that gout is associated with high intelligence. (I have not heard this theory propounded in connection with its preponderance among males, but the implication is there, as any woman can see!) There are enough brilliant names among the sufferers to give some credence to this theory, it is true, and some investigators have reported that people with gout tend, by and large, to have somewhat above average intelligence. They have even dug up explanations for this postulated "fact" in that the purines are among the important chemicals involved in brain function.

Other observers, however, express their doubts of any link between gout and mental prowess, some of them frankly scoffing at the idea. One rheumatologist is quoted thus: "In some patients, high levels of uric acid are better explained on the basis of high alcohol intake than on the basis of dazzling intellectual brilliance." Or it may simply be that in the past, the better educated segment of the population was also the most affluent, and had more frequent access to gout-stimulating food and drink.

Although researchers have not yet found a cure for gout, they have accomplished the next best thing by devising treatment schedules that keep it under control; that is, treatment can abort a current attack and to some extent ward off others.

The classical drug in the treatment of gout has been colchicine, a derivative of colchicum, one of the oldest drugs known, dating back thousands of years. It is reputed to be the poison brought by Medea from Colchis, hence its name. It has been continued throughout this time with varying amounts of enthusiasm, because of its possible toxic side effects. It can have a marked effect on gout, but little or none on other forms of arthritis. For this reason it is sometimes useful as a diagnostic agent. If an arthritic joint gets better with colchicine, the disease almost has to be gout. For centuries no one had a very good idea how colchicine works. Now there is a detailed explanation, as yet only a hypothesis, but supported by a logical sequence of events. It seems that colchicine restrains the white blood cells from cooperating in the vicious circle that effects the precipitation of more and more uric acid crystals.

In brief, the process goes something like this. One of the chief functions of the white blood cells is to act as a scavenging police force to keep the body as free as possible of harmful substances, by gobbling up such irritants anywhere they find them. For some reason, however, they are not able to engulf these uric acid crystals with impunity. The white cells suffer in the process and retaliate by releasing irritating substances in the immediate area, which increase the acidity of that area, which in turn, causes the precipitation of more uric acid crystals and so on, in the buildup of painful, swollen gouty joints. Just what does the colchicine do, then? One can only surmise, but in such a case the simplest explanation is often the correct one. Since a mere calming down of the white cells, making them a little less easily roused to active antagonism, would accomplish the purpose, that is most likely what the colchicine does. The use of this drug has to be monitored carefully, as it can have some unpleasant side effects, such as abdominal cramps and diarrhea.

Several other drugs have specific uses in gout, some that tend to prevent the overproduction and accumulation of uric acid. In addition, most of the drugs useful in other forms of arthritis are occasionally found beneficial in gout. One exception, and an unusual one in any kind of pain, is aspirin. Gouty patients may be given aspirin, but in more limited amounts.

The success of some of the newer drugs in the treatment of gout has greatly increased their use in recent years. Phenylbutazone is the most notable of these. Others are oxyphenbutazone and indomethacin. Still another, probenecid, is in a category of its own. It has no direct effect on the pain of gout, but increases the excretion of uric acid through the kidneys, thus helping to prevent the formation of the irritating uric acid crystals.

That time-worn order, "plenty of fluids," is well advised for gout, also. The logic of it seems self-evident. When there is a subversive substance in the body that tends to precipitate out and cause trouble when in too concentrated a solution, the sensible thing to do is to keep it well diluted.

Kidney disease is by far the most important complication of gout, and deaths reported from gout are usually from this complication. In any case of gout, the function of the kidneys is always kept under close observation and when kidney disease does occur, it must be treated as a separate entity. Drugs in use for the gouty joints would do nothing for the kidneys; in fact, some of these drugs are themselves a kidney hazard and require close supervision of the kidney function while they are being used on their own account.

4

Rheumatoid Arthritis

Nothing about the study of rheumatoid arthritis has been easy, and the primary problem has been the establishment of boundaries for it, getting it dissected out of the welter of associated diseases—rheumatic fever, gout, osteoarthritis, to mention a few of the most common ones—and set in a framework of its own, as a distinct disease entity. This has now been established to the satisfaction of most rheumatologists, although the boundaries remain blurred in a few areas. Cases crop up occasionally in which there is some fuzziness of diagnosis, cases that seem indisputably rheumatoid arthritis, yet overlap disturbingly into one of these other disease areas. In a few of these, there seems no other conclusion but that the two diseases are co-existent.

However, a few pinpoints of dissatisfaction with our entire system of grouping and nomenclature of

35

what we now call the rheumatoid diseases continue to exist in some quarters. Some persist in looking hopefully for an entirely new approach, one that will support more scientific precision in characterizations. One alternative that has been suggested is the use of the collagens, or connective tissue diseases, as the title umbrella under which to place rheumatoid arthritis, as it has attributes in common with others of this group. (Collagen is the protein that causes the water in which a soup bone has been boiled to become gelatinous upon cooling.) Most rheumatologists, however, are of the opinion that there are as many inexact areas in this grouping as in any other, that the only solution to the problem rests upon the identification of an indisputable common cause, whereupon rheumatoid arthritis and all the seemingly related diseases will automatically group themselves in their proper niches.

All this cloudiness as to cause and definition of rheumatoid arthritis carries over into its behavior. It is one of the most unpredictable of diseases. In the descriptions of diseases in medical textbooks, the "mode of onset" is always one of the categories discussed. Rheumatoid arthritis has its textbook "mode of onset" which it follows—sometimes. Almost as often it does not. This pattern (if one is justified in calling it that) consists of a low-grade fever, fatigue, loss of appetite, aching, joint pains. If the joint pains are severe or accompanied by swelling, the possibility of rheumatoid arthritis as a diagnosis is considered from the beginning. Otherwise the clinical picture is that of any type of low-grade infection, of either virus or bacterial origin, which gives an almost endless range of possibilities.

This mode of onset in itself shows endless variations. The beginning may be so insidious that by the time definite joint symptoms appear, the patient may have gotten over this vague, unexplained illness he had months or even a year or two before, which he probably called an attack of flu. Sometimes a patient feels certain that he never had any such acute episode, that the aching shoulder or knee or the swollen ankle came on him out of the blue, without any premonitory symptoms or signs. In which instance he probably comes in with his own diagnosis: "I've got arthritis, Doc. Think they'll ever find a cure for it?"

One case in which the onset seems rather dubious is that of a woman with severe rheumatoid arthritis who states that her trouble started when she was in her late forties, with no remissions worth speaking of. When she was twenty-nine, however, she had an attack of rheumatic fever during which both knees were badly swollen. Shortly after this she had a tonsillectomy. She had no more rheumatic fever, she states, and she never had any signs of trouble in her heart. The question that would arise in the minds of present-day rheumatologists is, "Was this really rheumatic fever, or was it her first attack of rheumatoid arthritis?"—a question impossible to answer at the time she had it, and only a matter of surmise now.

The majority of patients seem to strive for some degree of nonchalance about these early symptoms, trying to accept them as one of the penalties of aging. "Oh, well, after sixty it's all downhill," one woman told me when she came in using a cane for the first time.

When the beginning symptoms are vague, as they so often are, the effect on the patient may be more annoying than startling. The morning stiffness, the diffuse aches, seem like trials that one must put up with as one gets older, surely nothing to worry about. When the introductory sign is something that hampers activity, it is apt to be taken more seriously. Getting up in the morning and having to limp to the bathroom, finding that the "crick" in the knee does not go away and that one has to keep on limping down the stairs, can provoke the rebellious thought: "This is ridiculous! This can't be happening to me! Why, I'm in perfect health!"

Sudden involvement of a shoulder can be just as bad, when a woman finds that she can scarcely comb her hair in the morning. Routine questions I ask a woman in appraising the pathology in a shoulder are "Can you comb your hair?" and "Can you tie your apron?"

To some patients, the diagnosis of arthritis is a shattering pronouncement, almost unendurable. These are invariably people who have known someone with the disease in its most severe form, with the pain, crippling, and deformities that accompany advanced destructive changes in the joints. There is no nonchalance about these patients' attitudes nor do they volunteer any mention of the dread word "arthritis." What they are seeking frantically is some other explanation for their joint pains. As far as arthritis is concerned, they are in the denial stage. Any other diagnosis would be preferable, and some of them look until they find some doctor who, happily, offers them a substitute word, such as "bursitis" or "synovitis." Statistical facts afford them little reassurance. However small a minority these severe cases of arthritis are, they are the only ones with which these panicky patients can identify. The doctor who supplies an alternate diagnosis has little fear that he will be pinned down by embarrassing questions, such as "What's the difference between synovitis and

arthritis?" These patients are not looking for the truth
—rather for an escape from it. Let sleeping dogs lie;
sufficient unto the day is the evil thereof. Don't look at
it, and it may go away. These are the tenets of their
philosophy.

"Remissions" is the blessed word in arthritis. They
are the rule in this disease, more common here than
in any other. I have had patients recover from an acute
attack and tell me that it was almost worth the suffering
to realize how wonderful it is to be free of it. Perhaps
the patient in a mental institution who told a visitor that
he kept hitting himself on the head with a hammer
because it felt so good when he quit might not have
been any more crazy than a lot of other people.

While enjoying the bliss of a remission, it is easy for
a patient to believe that the disease is cured, that whatever he did for it was at last the magic formula. Patients
knowledgeable about arthritis, however, know that although remissions are the rule, so are recurrences.
"You never get the arthritis out of your body; it just
moves around to different places" is apt to be the
gloomy observation of an old sufferer, with a bulk of
historical fact to support him.

What to do to avoid another attack is hard to say,
since no one knows for sure what caused the first one.
In the face of all this ignorance, however, one precau-
tion seems sound on both a scientific and a commonsense basis—avoiding all possible strain or injury to the
diseased part. Any area of the body that has already
suffered some damage from disease is especially vulnerable to further trauma, and it seems only logical to
assume that this should be especially true of the joints.

As long as the pain and stiffness are present, a patient needs no other reminder not to overtax the

diseased joints, but when the remission is seemingly complete and the patient feels "as well as ever," it is easy to forget the rules of caution. One patient of mine was a hardworking farm wife whose living code did not permit her to omit any of her usual activities as long as she was physically able to carry on. So when her swelling and pain remitted sufficiently, she resumed scrubbing floors on her damaged knees, and taxed the joints of her back, elbows, shoulders, and hands with the hoeing and weed-pulling in her garden. These ill-advised activities must surely have contributed to her having become severely crippled in her old age.

The joint symptoms of rheumatoid arthritis are the ones the patient is most acutely aware of, sometimes to the complete exclusion of any others, and it may be only the doctor's questioning that brings others to mind in any detail or clarity. This is a systemic disease, one in which the entire body is involved. Among the general symptoms, less dramatic than those in the joints, may be weakness, fatigue, anemia, loss of appetite and weight. The hands and feet may be cold and sweaty. Sometimes there is numbness of the toes. Muscles, especially those in the area of the affected joints, are apt to be stiff and aching. Many of these symptoms are vague and tend to come and go, so that the patient is aware of "good days" and "bad days." Most patients will testify that weather has a marked effect on the way they feel, that they do not need to look at a barometer to be aware of impending weather changes.

Careful investigation in many areas outside the joints may often uncover lesions attributable to rheumatoid arthritis. Nodules may appear in almost any part of the body. Those under the skin are quite easily detectable, but those in the deeper tissues may escape notice unless they interfere with body function and cause signs and symptoms, such as pleural effusion and heart block. One such nodule has been identified as the center of a lesion causing thrombosis in a blood vessel.

The most common vascular accompaniment of rheumatoid arthritis is an inflammation in the walls of the smaller blood vessels. Many of these do not give any clinical signs, but the worst ones do. They are responsible in part for the coldness of the hands and feet of many arthritics, and they may be bad enough to cause ulcers in the calf of the leg, or gangrene of fingers and toes. This vasculitis may occur with other forms of arthritis, also. I know a patient with gouty arthritis who had to have a leg amputated because of gangrene.

Ulcerative colitis occurs in a notable number of cases of rheumatoid arthritis. There is some disagreement about the interpretation of this. Some think it is a coincidental occurrence, but the bulk of present opinion leans toward a definite relationship between the two diseases, even to the extent of adding a new member, colitic arthritis, to the already huge family of arthritides. One study strongly emphasizes the direct relationship between colitis and joint symptoms, citing a group of 151 patients with ulcerative colitis who were treated by removal of the entire colon. None of these developed arthritis, or had any recurrence of a previously existing joint disease. Arthritic patients occasionally develop a gastric ulcer, but this is sometimes an unfortunate side effect of drugs used in treatment.

Inflammation of the sheaths covering the nerves is an important complication of rheumatoid arthritis, and sometimes a very serious one. The nerves supplying the arms and legs are most commonly involved. More cases occur in women than in men, but men are more apt to develop the severe form. These lesions may cause clumsiness in the use of the extremities, numbness, diminution of sensation. Weakness and wasting of the muscles may follow. This inflammation along the sheaths of nerves may escape notice for a time, the pain being confused with that of adjacent sore joints. Another source of confusion is the difficulty of distinguishing between nerve entrapment conditions and inflammation along the nerve trunks themselves. In other words, it is possible for swollen or deformed joint structures to press upon a healthy adjacent nerve and cause pain similar to that of inflammation. Nerves emerging from the spinal cord are especially vulnerable to this type of injury from arthritic vertebrae.

Anemia is the most common nonarticular feature of this disease, varying in degree with its severity. Eye lesions are the next most common finding outside the joints. Many of these are mild, amounting only to a superficial inflammation of the conjunctiva, with some stickiness and grittiness at the lid margins. Deeper and more serious inflammation may occur, however, followed by ulceration or formation of cataracts.

Psoriasis occurs in a notable number of patients with rheumatoid arthritis, giving rise once again to the same old questions about the relationship between the two. Should either be considered a symptom of the other, or should another disease entity, psoriatic arthritis, be added to the list? It already has such a listing in the writings of some rheumatologists.

With this long train of possibilities attached to rheumatoid arthritis, it is easy to see how confusing it has been to define, and how impossible to predict. The best summarization of its course that I have read is that given by Harvard's Dr. Charles L. Short: "The course may be summarized as usually one of steady or intermittent progression, although complete or nearly complete remissions may occur at first and certain patients recover without significant disability even after years of active disease."

A more flippant summary might well be, "In this disease, anything can happen."

5

Arthritis in Childhood

A discussion of the ways in which arthritis can affect children makes the saddest chapter in any book on arthritis. Not that parents should be plunged into despair when a child develops arthritis; many young victims do well and recover without serious damage. My reason for opening on an ominous note is to emphasize that arthritis in childhood should be regarded from the beginning as a very serious disease, and that in order to minimize the possible tragic consequences, there should be no delay in seeking an accurate diagnosis and medical direction in treatment and care.

Only two diseases occur commonly enough to warrant discussion in this group: rheumatic fever and juvenile rheumatoid arthritis, both systemic diseases of a grave nature. The joint symptoms of rheumatic fever, however, are only secondary to more serious possible pathology elsewhere, usually in the heart. The arthritis usually clears up and is, in fact, little more than an alarm that may first call attention to the existence of rheumatic fever. In this respect it might be considered a benign occurrence, in that an early recognition of rheumatic fever predisposes a favorable outcome. Once this diagnosis is established, it also pinpoints the causative organism—the streptococcus, against which we have effective antibiotic weaponry. Also, the patient's heart will be kept under strict surveillance with preventive care against its involvement, or if cardiac involvement has already occurred, a prompt regimen of treatment is instituted. In effect, rheumatic fever is included in the group of arthritic diseases simply because arthritis is one of the findings, making its listing here an academic necessity. For all practical purposes of treatment and follow-up care, it belongs to the cardiologists.

Rheumatology or cardiology? From the viewpoint of responsibility, the pediatrician sees them as the same. An editorial in the *Journal of the American Medical Association* had this prodding title: "Is Rheumatic Fever Necessary?" With the cause established and the infective agent identified, it asks, why has it not been abolished, as have diphtheria and polio? Striving to be fair, the author then cites the peculiar difficulties that are present in the case of rheumatic fever. An effective immunization program is hampered by the fact that there are a multitude of kinds of streptococcus, and hypersensitivity reactions have followed intensive inoculation procedures. Since a natural attack of rheumatic fever fails to confer immunity, obtaining immunity by artificial means guarantees some difficulty.

A survey of the progress made against rheumatic fever in the past fifty years makes the present picture much less gloomy, however. A statement by that eminent physician, Sir William Osler, "Recognition of rheumatic fever is usually easy," means to present-day physicians that a great many cases were being overlooked. The pediatrician Emmett Holt said of it, "It is a disease of urban life; it is relatively infrequent in good homes"—a statement which few physicians could not contradict from their own case records. All agree that poverty with its attendant crowding is a large factor in its incidence, but few would fail to consider its possibility in the most affluent settings.

Juvenile rheumatoid arthritis is sometimes called Still's disease after George Frederick Still, who wrote the first clinical description of that disease before he was thirty years old. This description was his graduation thesis, written for his M.D. degree from Cambridge, a brilliant beginning of a career that went on to produce other works of value to medicine, among them a history of pediatrics.

Dr. Still's thesis, written in 1896, describes three types of rheumatoid arthritis that may occur in children. Hitherto there had been no classification made of juvenile arthritic disease. His work was based on cases he studied at the London Hospital for Sick Children, and it remains a classic among treatises on arthritis.

A typical picture cited by Dr. Still is that of an active, happy, apparently healthy four-year-old girl whose mother noticed one day that her daughter's knees seemed enlarged and that she appeared to move rather sluggishly in the mornings. She had not complained of pain and had had no other premonitory signs of illness. Her knees continued to enlarge further, and she had some swelling in her wrists and some stiffness

47

in her neck. Motion in her joints became markedly restricted, still without much apparent pain, and the muscles about her knees and wrists looked shrunken, wasted. By the time she came under the doctor's observation, her lymph glands and spleen were enlarged, and she was having periods of fever and sweating. As the disease progressed, other joints became involved. A remarkable development was that the child's growth was stunted, without, however, any mental deterioration.

Most of Dr. Still's cases were of the type just described. Another group showed similar joint symptoms, with no enlargement of the spleen or lymph nodes. In a third group there was the same joint stiffness, but the joint enlargement was in the form of fibrous nodules over the tendons. This type came to be described by some observers as chronic fibrous rheumatism.

Unfortunately for reasons of clarity, Still's disease has come to be defined variously. Some reserve the name for those cases of juvenile arthritis that come on abruptly, with fever; others for the cases in which there is enlargement of the spleen and lymph nodes. Some use the term much more loosely to mean any arthritic disease of childhood.

This juvenile form of rheumatoid arthritis is not a common disorder, and it is rarely fatal. It can, however, cause severe crippling, and thus leads to the slow accumulation of crippled adults. As with other arthritic diseases, the usual intensive studies have been made to determine the relationship of this disease to the others in the group. These studies appear to support the view that the rheumatoid arthritis of adults and children is a single entity.

In children, the onset is usually below the age of

five years, sometimes as early as six months. It may make its first appearance as an acute illness but a diagnostic puzzle, with a high fever, rash, and generalized aching, even with some pericarditis or pleurisy, the joints being uninvolved until a later stage. In other patients the first sign is arthritis, which may involve a number of joints simultaneously; or only one joint may be involved, often a knee. In a few cases, one of the extra-articular signs such as eye inflammation may appear first, with the arthritis delayed until weeks or months later. As has been stated, some patients make a good recovery, but in any case of this disease there are the dire possibilities of permanent crippling, blindness, or death.

"We know everything about rheumatoid arthritis except its cause and cure," was the sardonic remark made by one rheumatologist. Our "in-between" knowledge, makes the picture somewhat brighter, however; brighter to the extent that with early diagnosis and treatment, an estimated seventy to eighty percent of patients with juvenile rheumatoid arthritis achieve excellent functional status, and almost two thirds enjoy complete remission. Admittedly, this still leaves a tragic number of the 175,000 afflicted children in the United States in the dark side of the picture, a pressing incentive to research the cause and ultimate prevention of this disease.

The eye inflammation, iritis, that sometimes accompanies rheumatoid arthritis appears to be not very well known to the general public, although it has been recognized as a possible development by physcans since the early 1800's. One of the earliest of such cases to be reported was that of William Hickling Prescott in 1815, who survived his afflictions to become the leading historian of his day. His case history makes a medical suspense story. When he was nineteen years old he was stricken with a severe inflammation in his right eye. It appeared to be a conjunctivitis, and his doctors treated it as such according to the lights of that day, with leeches, lotions, blistering of the skin, purges, and bleedings. The condition became steadily worse, and by the end of a week he had lost the sight in the eye. (This was his good eye; he had been permanently blinded in his left eye two years before, when accidentally hit in the eye by a piece of bread thrown in the Commons hall at Harvard.) About a week later the joint symptoms of rheumatoid arthritis began. The knees and varying smaller joints were involved. His subsequent history is one of incapacitating illness from his arthritis, during which intervals his sight was restored temporarily. Then more eye inflammation blinded him again for a time. In the midst of these agonizing buffetings of illness, he submitted his first historical essay for publication. It was rejected. As any writer will understand, this must have been the nadir of discouragment for him. He suffered throughout the rest of his life from recurrences of these joint and eye symptoms, to which was added some digestive trouble thought to have been ulcerative colitis. He kept a strict work schedule for himself, however, having a secretary read to him during the times when his sight failed. He died of a stroke at sixty-three.

Medical historians draw an interesting parallel between the life of Prescott and that of Francis Parkman, who lived a generation later. Both were Bostonians who attended Harvard and were elected to Phi Beta Kappa. Both were trained in law, but were prevented from practicing their profession because of incapacitation by arthritis and poor eyesight. Each became a writer and the leading historian of his era.

This historical data may seem extraneous to the subject under discussion, but it is included here with a distinct therapeutic purpose in mind. Helpful treatment is not all medicine and surgery. Sometimes an uplift to the spirit accomplishes wonders, and nowhere is there a greater need for it than in such a chronic torturing disease as arthritis. It is hoped that the accomplishments of these two men under the most adverse circumstances may be an inspiration to other sufferers.

The clinical facts about a case of juvenile rheumatoid arthritis as related in any scientific writing give only the bare unemotional skeleton of such a tragedy as it exists in an afflicted family, affecting all its members. Talking to the parents of such a child makes it possible to visualize the damaging and destructive effects—physical, mental, and emotional—of this disease on a heretofore healthy, bright, attractive, perhaps gifted child, and their permeation throughout all aspects of the family life. It is not a story to which one can listen unmoved.

The illness of one such child started when she was a year and a half old. There is one older and one younger child in the family, both healthy. This little girl walked at the age of eleven months. When she was a year and a half old, her parents noticed that she was limping, favoring the left leg. They were not seriously concerned at first. "Oh, she's probably bumped herself," they said. "She's such a wild little rascal, into everything." They could find no bruise or sore spot on the leg, however, and she continued to limp. When her knee became swollen, they took her to a doctor.

"We hadn't thought of arthritis," the mother said;

"didn't know babies that young got it. And her knee never pained her much. She never has had much pain with her arthritis. To this day, we have never had to give her any pain medicine but aspirin, and not a lot of that."

For the next few years this little girl's knee was a major problem in this family, financial as well as medical. There were frequent trips to the orthopedists at university hospitals. Contractures of the tendons about the joint occurred, so that the leg could not be straightened, necessitating surgery. Growth of the left leg was impaired. Leg braces needed to be fitted and kept properly adjusted. "We go as clinic patients; we could never in the world afford to pay full price for everything we have had done. And even at that, it costs us plenty, by the time we travel to Iowa City and stay a few days, and pay somebody to look after the children at home."

This girl is now fifteen years old. Trouble with her eyes started about five years ago. Her parents and teachers noticed that her vision seemed impaired. She was holding her book closer and closer in order to read. Cataracts have developed in both eyes, attempts at prevention having been unavailing. Her parents have had to accept help from the association for the blind. She attends school, but does her study by listening instead of reading, her lessons having been taped for her. Her mother is kept busy on school days getting her transported to and from classes. The mother retains an admirable amount of optimism, which must surely be a sustaining strength to the child. The ophthalmologists encourage the hope that after several more years one or both eyes may have vision restored by surgery.

This girl's knee has been the only joint involved in

her arthritis, and it has been quiescent for some time. "We don't pay much attention to her arthritis any more," the mother told me. "Maybe we should, but her eyes have taken all our worry and time and attention for the past several summers. I don't know how we could have crowded anything else in—or paid for it, either."

The mother touched briefly upon the terrible cruelty of other children. The savage laughter of classmates when someone trips an almost sightless child, causing her to fall and let her books go scattering. The coarse epithets hurled at her, under the mistaken protection of anonymity. "They think I don't know who they are because I can't see them," she tells her mother, "but I always know their voices." Which is more deeply wounded in such instances, mother or child?

Her emotional strains have increased greatly in the past year, with the growth of romantic boy-girl relationships among her classmates. Schisms are occurring between her and girls who have been her good friends because of this development of an unshared interest. The time may come when she will have compensations for this void in her life. I have seen it happen. But that is little solace to a teen-ager.

6

Ankylosing Spondylitis

The rather ponderous title of this disease is sometimes shortened to its initials, AS. It is also called Marie-Strümpell disease (Marie Strümpell, by the way, is not the name of a lady, but a compound of the names of two male investigators). An old designation, "rheumatoid spondylitis," has been discarded as suggesting an erroneous identification with rheumatoid arthritis.

As is true with many other scientific designations, the name ankylosing spondylitis is a useful one, being properly descriptive of the nature of the disease. "Ankylosing" means fixing, making immovable, stiffening, cementing into place. "Spondylitis" means inflammation of the vertebrae. Thus the name alone cites the salient points of the disease, an inflammation of the vertebrae that results in fixation of parts or all of the spine. "Pokerspine" is another name used to describe this condition.

Although this disease shows itself most prominently and consistently in the spinal column, it is by no means limited to this area. Since its effects may be widespread, ankylosing spondylitis must be classified as a systemic disease. There may be arthritis in other joints, and eye inflammation, iridocyclitis, is found to be a complication in almost a third of all cases. Cardiovascular pathology is sometimes present—valvular insufficiency, enlargement of the heart, and pericarditis. A frequent association has been noted between ankylosing spondylitis and ulcerative colitis, regional enteritis and psoriasis, for none of which any logical explanation has been found. It is usual and sensible for investigators of any of the group of arthritic diseases to continue probing for possible connections with the others. Who knows when some missing link may not prove to be the obscure triggering device for the whole execrable lot of them? Following this line of research, some indications have been found suggesting a connection between this disease and juvenile rheumatoid arthritis.

Ankylosing spondylitis, like gout, is predominently a man's disease, said to attack men ten times as often as women. A case that remains prominently in my mind, however, is that of a pretty and charming young matron who had the disease primarily in the cervical portion of her spine. To turn her head she had to twist her entire body about. Because the onset is most commonly between the ages of fifteen and thirty-five, a group of California investigators, Drs. John J. Calabro, Bertram A. Maltz, and Paul Sussman have called this the most frequently overlooked cause of backache in young men.

The disease may begin, but rarely, with arthritis in the knees, hips, or ankles, or with recurrent eye inflammations. By far the most common beginning symptom is backache, estimated to occur in about sixty-five percent of the cases. This is described as a pain low in the back, which may be quite severe, and apt to occur at night. The patient has some stiffness when he first gets up, but this usually wears off as he moves about. He may also have some fatigue, loss of appetite and of weight, and slight fever.

As the disease progresses, a whole train of other symptoms sets in, directly traceable to the spreading involvement of the intervertebral joints. In the chest, the joints between the vertebrae and the ribs become affected. The patient can no longer expand his chest for efficient breathing and must learn to use his diaphragm. The inflammation about the joints may increase to the point of impinging on the nerves as they exit from the spinal cord, causing radiculitis or sciatica. All this causes pain, not all of which is in the joints. The muscles about the affected joints tighten up in a protective sympathy as muscles always do about an inflamed spot, and as a result they too get sore from the prolonged contraction. In an attempt to ease this combined pain of sore joints and muscle spasm, the patient often hunches over into any position he finds least intolerable, with the inevitable result that the back becomes distorted out of its normal shape.

After a suggestive history of backache in a young man, the first steps the physician makes toward a diagnosis are in the examining room. A number of simple tests are helpful. Determination of the chest expansion is one. An expansion of less than five centimeters is considered highly suggestive of arthritic disease in the joints between ribs and vertebrae. Inability to touch the floor, while keeping the knees straight, is presumptive evidence of disease in the lumbar spine. To test involvement of the vertebrae of the neck, the patient is required to place his heels and back against the wall. If his cervical spine is free from disease, he should be able to touch the wall with the back of his head, without raising his chin above carrying level. A suspected diagnosis may be confirmed by X ray.

No kind of radiotherapy is advised as treatment, however, because of the danger of leukemia. Acute myelogenous leukemia, as long as fifteen years after the therapy was stopped, has been reported in some of these cases. The usual regimen of treatment begins with drugs to relieve the pain and discomfort to the point where the patient can tolerate physiotherapy, and then an individualized combination of these two approaches. Aspirin, in the highest dosage tolerated, is the first choice of drugs, but it sometimes needs to be replaced or supplemented by some of the other anti-arthritic medications. Choice by trial and error is the rule here.

These are the mere basics of treatment, to which each physician adds his own individual refinements. Long-time care is required, at intervals that insure proper supervision to guard against further deformities, and all possible improvement of the old ones. Advice about posture, rest, sleeping arrangements, and exercises are helpful. No small part of the treatment is the bolstering of the patient's morale, best done by enabling him to see the improvements being made, however small. No patient with ankylosing spondylitis should feel that his case is hopeless. With well-directed effort, most victims can achieve happy, useful lives.

58

7

Less Common Diseases
in the Arthritic Group

Several of the so-called arthritic diseases have so much involvement with connective tissue that there may be a question as to where the predominant pathology exists. It is to this group that some investigators have given the name of the previously mentioned collagen diseases. The word "collagen" refers to the albuminoid substance present in the white fibers of connective tissue, in cartilage and in bone. Thus the term "collagen disease" does appear to be more inclusive than "arthritis," and the more radical adherents to this terminology would prefer this title to that of "arthritic disease." The most recent tendency, however, is to place under the collagen title only those diseases in which connective tissue involvement usually predominates.

Scleroderma is one of these. The word means "hardened skin," which is descriptive of its most prominent feature, the thickening and hardening of variable areas of skin. This is only the surface manifestation of the disease, however. It is a serious affliction, and many internal organs may be involved, as well as numerous joints. It can occur at any age, but starts most often in the forties and fifties, more often in women than in men. Its behavior is as unpredictable as that of other arthritic diseases, progressing rapidly in some patients, and in others dragging along for years with many static intervals. Its seriousness depends upon the involvement of vital organs, which may include the lungs, heart, or kidneys. No treatment has been successful, or even very encouraging.

Perhaps the most important of this small and exclusive group of collagen diseases has the cumbersome title of systemic lupus erythematosus, usually referred to by its initials, SLE. It is important because it is a disease with frequent serious involvement of vital organs, notably the kidneys, and because its diagnosis has often been overlooked. Now, with more specific blood tests, it is possible to recognize cases that were formerly not recognized at all, or only after long delays. In some patients there may be such a long-drawn-out chronicity that only a symptom or two may exist for as long as ten or twelve years before the disease becomes full-blown with recognizable clinical signs.

These early symptoms may be indecisive and nonspecific—such things as anemia, or arthritis, which exist in the great majority of these cases. The skin signs, when they appear, are of more help in diagnosis. A typical picture is that of an inflammation on the face so violent as to resemble erysipelas. It is apt to extend from one cheek to the other, across the bridge of the nose, in a butterfly pattern.

SLE may occur at any age, but most frequently in

the twenties and thirties, and it attacks more women than men, in the proportion of five to one. As with other diseases of this sad group, there is no known cure. Chronic discoid lupus is a comparatively benign form of this disease.

Erythema nodosum is a disease of this group that has never stirred up much excitement in the medical world. Although it has been recognized for some time—Sir William Osler wrote about it over fifty years ago in his medical text for students, as a well-established entity—no one has ever discovered anything very bad about it. Its typical manifestation is the appearance of areas of reddish, slightly tender bumps on the skin, usually on the lower legs. They may last from several days to several weeks. The patient feels achy and fever-ish, has some muscle stiffness and malaise. Usually there is a story of pain in a variable number of joints which may have occurred several weeks before and disap-peared, or it may persist throughout the presence of the skin signs and for some time afterward. Occasion-ally a patient may regard the lumps as a visitation out of the blue, the joint pains having been so mild that he has forgotten them. That is not to say, however, that there is not some hidden thread yet to be identified, giving it a sinister connection with serious arthritic pa-thology. This happens repeatedly in medical research. Erythema nodosum may occur in a number of other serious diseases, including tuberculosis, but no causa-tive relationship has ever been established between these and arthritis with erythema nodosum. In one situation its presence may even be somewhat reassur-ing. Cases that offer a diagnostic problem because of other associated findings, in which it becomes impera-tive first to rule out malignancy (such as enlarged

61

lymph nodes, for example) get some bolstering encouragement with the appearance of erythema nodosum, since it is very rarely associated with malignant lesions.

As stated previously, this is not a worrisome disease, in the light of our present knowledge. It clears up completely without any serious aftereffects. It may come back, but recurrences are not common. If one had to suffer the visitation of some one of the arthritic diseases (and had any choice in the matter), this would be as good a one to pick as any.

The foregoing is by no means a complete list of the collagen diseases, only the more common ones. It may be well to repeat here that rheumatologists differ in their groupings of all these diseases, some of them including most of the arthritides under this title. For the purpose of this writing, however, only those diseases in which collagen dysfunction is predominant are included here.

To illustrate the depths of confusion sometimes associated with this subject, some rheumatologists deviate from the synonymous use of the terms "collagen" and "connective tissue." They recognize connective tissue diseases that are *not* of collagen origin, which arise in the elastic fibers of connective tissue, not the white ones that yield gelatin on boiling. These disorders, called elastica disease, are not commonly known, and are of no more than academic interest to the average lay reader.

Bursitis is an affliction most people have heard of, but it is not very well defined in their minds. It is often used as an alternate term to arthritis, as a name a little less common, and it is easy to see how well it lends itself to such use. A bursa is a small sac containing slippery fluid which acts as a cushioning device at potential friction points in a joint. It can become irritated and inflamed from pressure or injury, and the entire joint is apt to become red and swollen as a result. But where does the bursitis end and the arthritis begin? It happens most often to a shoulder, but may occur in other joints, notably hips or elbows, and it is treated in the same manner as other kinds of arthritis.

Bursitis may have a very sudden onset. One patient told me that she went to bed one night feeling perfectly well. When she woke in the morning she looked at the clock and noted that she would have to hurry to get to work on time, and nearly panicked when she found she could scarcely lift her right arm to fix her hair. She managed to do it with many contortions and by grimly enduring the pain in her shoulder, vowing that if this happened once more she would cut off her hair and buy a wig.

Another alternate term for arthritis, offering the same difficulties in distinction, is synovitis. It means an inflammation of the synovial membrane, which lines the joint capsule, and is thus a part of the pathology of most cases of arthritis.

Fibrositis is a term used sometimes, but with not much benefit. It is not even classified as a disease but is rather a name given to a group of unexplained symptoms (aches, pains, and stiffness, and is sometimes called "muscular rheumatism"—a rather misleading title as it seems to have no relation to other valid rheumatoid pathology, such as joint inflammation. It is an affliction of tense and nervous people, and not serious. It is important that an accurate diagnosis be made, however, ruling out organic rheumatoid disease.

It may be well to mention again in this discussion of the less common arthritides those kinds of arthritis

caused by specific types of infection. The most impor
tant of this group are those that follow tuberculosis,
meningitis, and gonorrhea. It is important to have as
prompt a diagnosis as possible in these cases, since the
treatment of each is the treatment of that particular
causative disease.

8

The Dozens of
Kissing Cousins

My definition of a kissing cousin is someone who greets
you with an embrace at a family reunion, whom you
remember only vaguely having heard of before, and
whom you are not apt to run across again and would
not recognize if you did.

Every large-scale textbook reunion will have a
chapter devoted to these kissing cousins of the arthritis
family. Most of the names in the chapter are known
chiefly in university circles and will be unfamiliar to
most readers. Some, quite properly, bear the name of
the university notables who fathered the research
about them, and thus, in effect, gave them birth. Others
have been christened more practically with names that
afford some clue to their origins or characteristics.
Some are not considered disease entities at all, and are
referred to merely as "syndromes" or clusters of findings.

These distant cousins are all interesting. Each of them elaborates in some way the basic knowledge of the family. While the names may be unfamiliar, a great many of us have doubtless seen some of these rarer members of the arthritis family, without knowing exactly what to call them. So, for expedience, we have diagnosed them as oddball members of whatever arthritis group with which they seem to have the most evident kinship. For example, one of these rare relatives known to the knowledgeable as palindromic rheumatism would doubtless go down in the records of any of the rest of us as a case of acute recurrent rheumatoid arthritis. (It would be all the same to the patient, since no one has mentioned curing any of these rarities.)

Palindromic rheumatism, was named for one of its chief characteristics, which is recurrence. "Palindromic" comes from a Greek stem, and means "tending to turn back," the same stem from which we named our noun "palindrome," which means something—a word, line, verse, etc.—that reads the same forward or backward. I cite this one from the dictionary: "Madam, I'm Adam."

Recurrence alone would not be reason enough to isolate this as a disease entity, since recurrence is a characteristic of other diseases of the group, notably of rheumatoid arthritis. It is the *frequency* of recurrence that is the outstanding feature. One series of cases studied reported an average of one hundred sixty-four attacks per patient in a seven-year period—which must not have allowed some of these patients very much time for recuperation between bouts.

Occasionally multiple joints are involved, but usually the disease attacks only one joint at a time, although it may move from one joint to another. When a toe joint has been the selected site, gout has been the first diagnosis to be considered, as the appearance of the joint and the excruciating nature of the pain is similar to that of gout.

There are some benign aspects of palindromic rheumatism: once the pain of the attack has been endured, that's it—that is, until the next attack comes. There is no damage to other parts of the body; the trouble is limited to the joints. Furthermore, the joints themselves suffer no permanent damage; there is no crippling. Truly this is one of the more benign forms of arthritis! But, alas, our satisfaction over this discovery is short-lived. No sooner was it established as a part of authentic arthritis data than some longer-term observers found that a considerable number of their cases developed rheumatoid arthritis later—too many to make the development a matter of coincidence. Now the weight of opinion is swinging toward the belief that these palindromic rheumatics are one form of an early stage of rheumatoid arthritis. So maybe palindromic rheumatism is not a kissing cousin, after all, but a maverick branch straight off the old family stock. All of which helps to keep the study of arthritis from becoming too boring.

Most readers are doubtless familiar with hemophilia, a chronic hereditary disease limited to the male sex, in which the clotting time of the blood is greatly prolonged, giving the patient a lifelong vulnerability to serious, even fatal, hemorrhage. A joint trouble these people may get is called, appropriately, hemophilic arthritis, and it is quite a common affliction among them, although it rates as one of the rare diseases in the general populace. It is caused by bleeding into a joint, most often the knee, sometimes the hip, ankle, shoulder, or elbow. Such bleeding may follow what seems to be a very slight injury. A prompt diagnosis is important, as the treatment differs from that of other forms of arthritis. Keeping an arthritic joint immobilized after the most acute pain has eased is taboo in most arthritis, but imperative here, to prevent further bleeding. If the doctor knows the patient and is aware that he has hemophilia, the diagnosis of the joint trouble will be no problem to him. In a patient with hemophilia, any sudden swelling anywhere is considered to be hemorrhage until proven otherwise. Sometimes in the early stages, the pain and pressure in the joint can be relieved most promptly by drawing out the blood with a syringe.

A number of other blood disorders have their typical accompanying joint syndromes. The first signs of leukemia, especially in children, may be pain and swelling in several joints, often accompanied by fever. A blood condition with a long name which means too little gamma globulin is sometimes complicated by joint signs that look like rheumatoid arthritis. (Rheumatoid arthritis has so many imitators that one wonders whether they can *all* be separate diseases.) Sickle cell anemia sometimes afflicts black children with joint involvement resembling rheumatic fever.

Several gastrointestinal diseases present worrisome side issues in the joints. There is a form of arthritis, for example, that "goes with" ulcerative colitis. For some years after it was first noted, it was thought to be rheumatoid arthritis occurring coincidentally in patients with ulcerative colitis, but later observers found a sufficient number of points of difference to believe it warrants classification as a separate disease. Ankylosing spondylitis is also a frequent complication of ulcerative colitis. Inflammatory disease of the small bowel, as well as the colon, may be accompanied by arthritis; also the symptom "steatorrhea" of unknown cause, characterized by the loss of undigested fat through the stools.

Structural abnormalities of the connective tissue give rise to a large assortment of joint diseases—a logical result since connective tissue is so important a component of joint structure. If the protective and supportive connective tissue of joint capsules fail to do what the joint depends upon, the result can be wobbliness of the joint to the point of insecurity of motion or support, the stringencies of contracture, or distortion of position of opposing joint surfaces. There are so many of these connective tissue dyscrasias that even a complete-appearing monograph such as that by E. G. L. Bywaters and Barbara Ansell states that they have omitted many. Some investigators claim there are upward of a hundred kinds of arthritis, which must include a preponderance of these syndromes related to connective tissue involvement. (What distinctions designate some of these as diseases and others as syndromes, I have not been able to determine. The terms appear to be used interchangeably.)

The name "gargoylism" was given to the earliest category of these connective tissue malformations to be described. As later investigators made more detailed studies, this original classification was found to be too broad, so names of other diseases and syndromes of the same general nature cropped up in the literature.

One notable study was made by Gertrud Hurler, a German pediatrician. Thus was born "Hurler's disease" or "Hurler's syndrome," as it appears in various texts, whose symptoms and signs make a horrendous picture in the aggregate. It is hereditary, and the onset is within the first two years of life. The typical appearance becomes established gradually, within the next four or five years. The head of the patient is large and bulging, the nose is flattened, the lips are protruding, the tongue is thickened, the facial features in general are coarsened. The teeth are apt to be small and widely spaced, often malformed, with swollen gums. There are marked changes in the vertebral column, the neck being shortened and the lower back humped. Joints of the extremities are involved also, resulting in fixation of the hip, elbow, shoulder, or knee, and clawing of the hands. The mentality of these patients is badly impaired; sometimes they are deaf and blind. The only halfway merciful part of their story is that they seldom live beyond the age of twenty.

Hunter's syndrome is similar to Hurler's, but not quite so bad. It develops more slowly, gives no mental retardation or eye trouble, and is limited to males. Morquio's disease is another growth anomaly which appears at about the age of two, with deformities first noted about the chest. The back becomes humped and the breastbone sticks out in front. These patients usually make no further growth after the age of ten. They become knock-kneed and flatfooted and have a waddling gait due to a combination of muscle weakness and joint capsules too lax to give good support.

This hypermobility of joints is a finding that runs through quite a number of this disease group, one of which, because of the exclusivity of this feature, is known as hypermobility syndrome. The Ehlers-Danlos syndrome is similar, but has an abnormal fragility of the skin in addition.

The outstanding sign of Marfan's syndrome is an elongation of the bones of the extremities, making the typical picture that of a tall, thin loose-jointed individual with particularly long fingers, a condition which has a name of its own, arachnodactyly, which means "spider fingers." (No mention is made as to whether it contributes anything to piano-playing skill.)

This dissertation could go on and on, with small profit to the reader. Few people who read this book will have suffered from any of the extremely rare diseases already listed, or known anyone else who did. It is just possible that a condition mentioned here will jar the reader to a first recognition of something he has seen.

9

What Deeply Hidden Roots?

There is no valid excuse for the medical profession's centuries of neglect in going all out against arthritis, but there is one important explanation. Arthritis is not a killing disease. It has always seemed more urgent to focus scientific attention on such things as diphtheria or poliomyelitis. What does another ten years or so matter to the arthritic? He will still be here. That ten years of torture may have been added to his life has not received due consideration.

The treatment of arthritis has been shunned by many doctors, mostly because of their own feeling of inadequacy. Achieving brilliant cures, and saving lives is much more satisfying to the ego, and arthritis is not the field for either of these. Sir William Osler, author of *Principles and Practice of Medicine,* which was the medical bible for my generation of students (and many before and after me), once admitted, "When an arthritis patient comes in the front door, I feel like going out the back door."

The amateur arthritis researchers may at first feel exuberant at the luxuriance of the field in which they have chosen to work. "What a wealth of material is all about us!" they exult. "No one could fail to learn a lot of new things here."

In a short time, however, their exultation may well change to groans. "What a jungle! How can I ever find my way through it, much less distinguish anything in it?"

Arthritis has always been a disease jungle. Osteoarthritis was the predominant overgrowth from early times, when it dictated the accepted picture of arthritis, that of a crippled and bent elderly figure. It was a concomitant of aging, and it existed everywhere. A long time elapsed before people began to look critically at the individual plants in this jungle, to note that they were not all exactly alike, that there were many variations and groups of variations, and that hidden among the tougher overgrowths were more fragile shoots that came in time to be given such names as rheumatic fever or Still's disease. Truly, the wealth of material, paradoxically, makes arthritis research more difficult.

The patient may be able to accept the fact of arthritis as an evil visitation, of which he is one of the unfortunate targets. But the physician knows that no disease "just happens," springs up from nowhere, not even in the vulnerable joints. It *has* to be the result of a logical, provable chain of events, and it is toward the identification of these that his questions turn. While answering a patient's questions with as much aplomb as we can muster, we are asking ourselves, why, after all these thousands of years, haven't we got the entire modus operandi of arthritis figured out?

When Editor Howard J. Sanders asked Dr. Theodore B. Bayles of Harvard Medical School, one of the nation's top authorities on rheumatic diseases, what he believed to be the most likely causes of rheumatoid arthritis, Dr. Bayles replied, "G.O.K.—God Only Knows!"

This is the kind of joke a doctor can make when he is feeling less witty than self-critical. It is a self-criticism that is shared to some extent by the entire profession.

Such statements, however, are explosions of frustration. To feel pessimistic about the recent progress and the present outlook in the entire field of rheumatology would be a denigration of the outstanding recent accomplishments. In research, it is always the "breakthroughs" that get the headlines, but behind each of these successes is a myriad of failures, many of which have contributed to the final success by nudging future investigators away from proven dead ends.

Albert Einstein's biographer, Ronald W. Clark, makes frequent allusions to Einstein's years-long search for a unified field theory, an equational meeting point for electromagnetics and gravitation. After spending six months on one such line of endeavor, he found that it was an erroneous approach, but he told a friend he planned to publish his results anyway, "To save another fool from wasting six months on the same idea."

Mankind's oldest disease is now truly in a stage of "rheumatism renewal," in the sense of research attention being paid to it. Philip Hench's definition of rheumatism is the best statement I know of the boundaries limiting such research: "Rheumatism is pain anywhere within half a mile of a joint." In other words, there are no anatomical limits to the possible encroachments of the rheumatoid family of diseases. Suspicion follows them everywhere. The literature now appearing is shot through with studies seeking a possible connection between members of the arthritis family and diseases that have heretofore been considered outsiders—as well as further connecting links between the family members themselves by way of cementing the relationships and reenforcing the basic family definition.

These studies have most frequently followed the routine of picking up some surface manifestation of the arthritic group of diseases, looking for any hint of it that may appear elsewhere, and trying to find a connection. Throughout the ages, inflammation of a joint or multiple joints has been the identifying bloom, the visible fruit, accepted common denominator for the entire group of diseases. At this stage of intensive study it is doubtful that any type of joint inflammation has escaped scrutiny. Any logical hint of a connection between arthritis and any other disease gets a full rundown by research groups.

The identification of other common denominators has already increased the boundaries of this family circle considerably. Mention has been made in other chapters of connective tissue involvement in some members of the arthritides group, and the suggested classification of "collagen diseases." Anything new discovered about arthritis gives rise to a flurry of enthusiasm as to where it will lead, what enlightenment it will afford on the known arthritic diseases, and what connections it may establish in other directions.

Out of this welter of unproven possibilities, one concept arises to greater and greature stature: that of the presence of some essential but as yet unidentified triggering mechanism. Suppose a group of investigators set out to analyze the make-up of a rifle cartridge or shotgun shell, never having seen one before, knowing only that it is capable of highly destructive action. Taking it from the box on a shelf where it may have lain for months, innocent-looking, inert, unchanging, pulling it apart and spreading its contents on the laboratory table, it is possible that they might have all the ingredients in plain sight and properly identified for some time before they realize that it is the final ping on the primer which changes the inertia to explosion. Rheumatoid arthritis seems just as mystifying, and it is not too far-fetched to consider that it may have a similar explanation.

In a disease which exhibits any kind of inflammatory reaction, infection must always be the prime suspect. This has been true of arthritis from the time anything was known about infectious organisms.

One of the oldest and most tenacious theories about the cause of arthritis is that of focal infection; that there are little pockets of pus hidden in obscure places in the body, most likely in the teeth or tonsils, which supply inflammatory material to new strongholds in the most vulnerable areas, such as the joints. A collateral finding in the arthritic Neanderthal man was that he had also had pyorrhea. A body disinterred in Rhodesia showed caries in the jaw, and erosions from abscesses in the maxillae. The Incas and Aztecs of the Americas suffered from arthritis to an unusual extent, and examination of their skulls reveal that they had had a great many abscesses at the root of their teeth. Observers have pointed out that these Indians had reached a high stage of civilization, whereas the less civilized Indians of the North had fewer bad teeth, and much less arthritis.

The medical history of Louis XIV appears to give credence to the focal infection theory of the cause of arthritis. After the decay and extraction of teeth, he had an acute inflammation of multiple joints and another severe bout with arthritis four years later, following the development of an anal fistula.

Ever since we have known about infection and its causative organisms, scientists have been digging for proof of an infectious cause for rheumatoid arthritis. To many of them it is the Lost Dutchman Mine in the hills of rheumatology. Some of them have become so carried away by their zeal that they have uttered premature cries of "Eureka!" on occasion, only to have their findings discredited later by other impartial, cold-blooded researchers.

Editor Howard J. Sanders, of *Chemical and Engineering News,* quotes Dr. John L. Decker, chief of the Arthritis and Rheumatism Branch of the National Institute of Arthritis and Metabolic Diseases, as follows: "If rheumatoid arthritis were produced by a common, easy-to-culture bacterium continually present in joints, the cause of this disease might very well have been discovered by Pasteur a hundred years ago. Obviously, things are not that simple." "Things are not that simple" is a statement with which no rheumatologist would disagree.

It is a proven fact that a few forms of arthritis are caused by infectious agents, and the agents have been identified, among them the streptococcus, staphylococcus, gonococcus, viruses, and other infective organisms.

These types of arthritis, however, are a minor category in the entire arthritic group, accounting for less than one percent of all cases—and an important fact to remember is that none of these are rheumatoid arthritis.

Thus it must be admitted that there was some sound foundation for the focal infection theory of the cause of arthritis, and it has still not been completely abandoned. But after the sacrifice of an incalculable number of innocent teeth and tonsils, we have been forced to the conclusion that the answer is not that simple. The focal infection theory may be a part of it, but not all.

However, cases such as the above make it easy to understand why the infections persist as a theoretical cause of rheumatoid arthritis as well. Other promising possibilities have come to light, then faded. This old theory seems to have too much going for it to be discarded entirely, in spite of lack of direct evidence. The general picture of the onset of rheumatoid arthritis is often similar to that of an infection—there may be inflammation, low-grade fever, lack of appetite, loss of weight, increased sedimentation rate of the red blood cells, increase in number of white blood cells—all of which are typical of an infectious process.

One rheumatologist has put his credo into an equation: "Arthritis equals infection plus x." Most present-day researchers are in agreement, although some of them would capitalize the x.

Among the ideas that gained some temporary ascendancy over the infectious theory was one that tied rheumatoid arthritis with hormonal imbalance. There is some valid support for the suspicion that arthritis could have a connection with hormone dysfunction. In the first place, there is a marked difference between the sexes in the incidence of arthritis. Women are almost three times as prone to develop rheumatoid arthritis as men. It has been noted, furthermore, that women suffering from the disease have noticed marked relief from symptoms during a pregnancy. A most significant finding followed the development of the adrenocortical hormones, cortisone and hydrocortisone, when it was noted that they have a strikingly beneficial ameliorative effect on the symptoms of arthritis.

With all this data to go on, it is not surprising that researchers turned down the hormone trail, confident of at last finding the elusive answer to the cause of arthritis. But their sniffings were to no avail. Each hormone-related fact proved to be an isolated entity, leading nowhere else, as far as they could discover. Nonpregnant women with arthritis obtained no benefit from the hormones known to be secreted in large amounts during pregnancy. No significant difference has been found between the level of adrenocortical steroids in patients with rheumatoid arthritis and those free from the disease. Most dismaying of all was the discovery that the remarkable relief that arthritic patients often obtain from steroids is relief from *symptoms* only, and not at all curative. Furthermore, the relief is only temporary, lasting only as long as the drugs are used, and the basic destructive processes of the disease are not affected.

Allergies have had their day in the search for possible causes of rheumatoid arthritis, but as intensive studies of these reactions have brought more enlightenment upon the allergies themselves, they have failed to establish any causative connection with arthritis.

Most researchers have now given up the idea that arthritis bears any relation to the spectrum of allergic reactions commonly recognized.

However, another phase of hypersensitivity, called autoimmunity continues to receive much scientific attention. The body's immune mechanism is a wonderfully protective force when in normal working order. It can be stimulated to form antibodies against harmful substances from the outside, thus making it possible to stamp out infectious diseases. In protective inoculations the body's immunizing system is stimulated to form such an overwhelming army of antibodies against that particular disease that none of the causative agents of that disease can ever get a foothold. These antibodies are never inactivated, usually give lifetime protection.

An autoimmune disease is one in which something has gone haywire with the body's immunizing system, causing it to manufacture antibodies against some of its own cells or their constituents. As one scientist explained it, "Civil war breaks out in the body itself." There are two main theories as to why this happens. One is that the immunizing system itself has lost some of its acuity, becoming defective in some way. Possible reasons given for this deterioration are aging, hereditary abnormality, metabolic defects, exposure to harmful outside agents such as bacteria, chemicals, or X rays. The other theory is that the immunizing system is in perfect working order, well able to distinguish normal from abnormal, but that the body of the rheumatoid arthritis patient is making abnormal changes in normal substances. The result is an evil chain reaction in which these abnormal substances are relentlessly attacked and destroyed, making the joints increasingly worse and the stimuli to destruction increasingly greater.

Although the workings of the autoimmune reaction is still a matter of theory, the actual existence of autoimmune diseases has much scientific credence. In fact, another of the rheumatic diseases, systemic lupus erythematosus, is believed to belong in this category. One form of inflammation of the thyroid gland, called Hashimoto's thyroiditis, is believed to be caused by these damaging autoantibodies. Some diseases, considered infectious in origin, are believed to be perpetuated by the body's autoimmune reaction. Suspicion of this kind of collusion between infection and autoimmunity is attached to leprosy and to rheumatic fever.

In the battle against the arthritic diseases, rheumatoid arthritis is the center of the target the researchers are aiming at. They believe that when its secrets are cracked open for scientific scrutiny, the mysteries of most of the others will be unfolded. Treatises on rheumatoid arthritis are dotted with such descriptive phrases as "a fascinating enigma," "most puzzling as to etiology," "a capricious disease of unknown cause, uncertain course, and variable prognosis."

One of the most sensational events in the research on rheumatoid arthritis was the discovery of the "rheumatoid factor," one of the gamma globulins believed by scientists to be an autoantibody. Proof of its presence in the serum of patients with rheumatoid arthritis was thought by many to be a direct indication that the disease is caused by autoimmune reaction.

Hopes were high for what it would do for diagnosis, prognosis, and classification of arthritic diseases. Here might be a test as specific for arthritis as the old Wassermann was considered to be for syphilis. But it did not turn out that way.

The subjects of autoimmunity and rheumatoid factor produced a series of reports of experiments and enthusiastic exposition of theories by hopeful investigators, which have been promptly shot down by other investigators, followed by other theories and demolitions, ad infinitum. In the late 1950's, for example, two investigators found two prisoners who consented to be the subjects of an experiment. The experiment was prolonged over a six-week period, during which time the subjects were transfused at intervals with rheumatoid factor in sufficient amounts to keep their concentration at a high level. Both subjects were free from arthritis at the beginning, of course, and neither developed it, giving rise to some investigators' rash conclusion that rheumatoid factor is harmless.

The experiment has been considered noteworthy, but not conclusive. Two subjects are too few on which to base conclusions. The rheumatoid factor had been present in their serum for a limited time, perhaps not long enough to provoke the development of symptoms. Some scientists believe that the rheumatoid factor, to be typically injurious, would have to be present within the synovial membrane and have some already-altered, and therefore abnormal, gamma globulin with which to react. In any case, rheumatoid factor was discovered to be present in the serum of patients with other diseases besides arthritis (tuberculosis, for one) as well as in apparently healthy elderly people—although usually not in such high concentration. Moreover, it is *not* present in all cases of rheumatoid arthritis.

As a result, the rheumatoid factor has been the subject of heated controversy for the past forty years, with no resolution yet in sight. What *has* been proved is merely the presence of the rheumatoid factor in the serum of many patients with rheumatoid arthritis. That it has any causative connection still remains in doubt. Many skeptics believe that it merely "goes with" the disease, but does not cause it. Some have gone so far as to think it is beneficial, being one of the defensive substances manufactured by the body to fight the disease.

The rheumatoid factor is still considered a valuable descriptive feature of rheumatoid arthritis—it appears to have a bearing on the projected severity of the attack —and it is quite likely that it has other values not yet determined, but it is not the decisive finding that was once hoped for.

In spite of all the controversy over rheumatoid factor, however, it is proving to be an adjunct to the work of researchers in several small ways. It adds one more descriptive bit to the disease profile. It is a diagnostic aid in that it gives us a fairly specific test for rheumatoid arthritis, since it is not present in significant amounts in any other form of arthritis. It throws some light on the outlook for a patient with rheumatoid arthritis. One with a low concentration of the rheumatoid factor in his serum is more likely to have remissions, while someone else with high concentrations is apt to have the severe form of the disease. These are generalities, however, which may have many exceptions. With the present marshaling of research forces against it, it seems a valid hope that rheumatoid arthritis is doomed to extinction.

Cogitations about the rheumatoid factor, however, have demonstrated in what varied directions the roots of a disease may lead—in this case, outside the human race entirely, into a number of animals. Some research thinkers, both medical people and veterinarians, noted that in some respects the rheumatoid factor is similar to a substance found in the serum of rats, poultry, swine, and sheep following mycoplasmal infections that have caused arthritis in these species. The diseases respectively are called mycoplasma arthritides, synovia, hyorhinus, and Bedsonia. In brief, the things we know about the rheumatoid factor are mostly hints, implications, possibilities, with nothing proved about its significance or its value. Its present aspect is that of an intense immune response to some chronic viral, bacterial, or mycoplasmal infection. But, intense as it is, it is still not powerful enough to kill off the infection. So what good is it? The biological purpose of an immune reaction is to kill off the enemy that provoked it. For all we know about it now, the rheumatoid factor is merely a passive piece of evidence.

Since the cause of rheumatoid arthritis has proved to be so elusive, the search for its identity has naturally led researchers to consider every known disease-causing mechanism. Backtracking along possible origins from the past offers endless possibilities of discovery. Single-mindedness of purpose has no place here. We do not know what we are looking for but wish to learn what there is to be found, keeping open minds as to where and in what form it may present itself. The gold we seek may be imbedded in any tissue in the body.

The stories patients tell about how their arthritis started are all worthy of consideration, but they do not prove anything. Some people feel certain that their joint trouble started at the time of some other illness, often an upper respiratory infection, or just as another illness was subsiding. Respiratory infections are so common, however, that coincidence in these cases has to be considered. On the other hand, there are people who attribute their arthritis to accidental injury, fatigue, emotional upset, or exposure to cold and dampness.

In the studies of Egyptian mummies it was noted that the percentage of those afflicted with arthritic joint changes was greater among the ones along the Nile than in the inhabitants of the more arid regions. One body disinterred from an Egyptian cemetery had such marked arthritic distortions of fingers and toes that it was questioned whether such severe pathology could have occurred in the benign climate of Egypt, whether this man was not a visitor from some more humid area in Asia.

It has been noted that the inhabitants of the far north, those coldest areas of human habitation, are the only people known who rarely if ever have arthritis except that which may be attributed to injury. They live half the year without sunshine, and their traditional diet is limited to meat, fish, and blubber.

Climate undoubtedly has an effect on the symptoms of many arthritic patients, but it is a very undependable source of relief. A great many patients are sensitive to the weather and can predict weather changes by the aches in their joints. A warm, dry climate is traditionally the kind favored by these patients, but it is nothing for them to bet on; especially to the extent of pulling up stakes and moving without first giving the new locale a trial. There are some patients who get no relief whatever in what is considered the perfect climate for them.

In the form of osteoarthritis which we call the secondary type, a cause-and-effect sequence is clearly in evidence. It usually follows injury to an adjacent joint, and the onset is apt to occur later in a patient's life than the primary type. This is the kind of osteoarthritis that may cause a patient to declare, "I never had any arthritis at all, to speak of, until I broke my leg that time, and this knee has bothered me ever since."

Since stress within the joint appears to be the important causative factor, it is easy to see how a fracture in one of the bones could contribute to it. Pain, defective alignment (even if only temporary), protective positioning of the extremity, anything that deflects the normal apposition of the bones of the joint to any degree, detracts from the smooth operation of that joint and becomes irritating. Hence the development of arthritis.

It has been estimated that ninety-seven percent of all people over sixty have osteoarthritis in some degree. This universality of occurrence among the aging gives credence to the belief that it is a natural accompaniment of the aging process. But it is never a very satisfactory scientific conclusion to say that any disease is simply caused by old age. It practically admits that there are some underlying factors, associated with the aging process, some hows and whys, being overlooked. One logical assumption is that heredity plays some part; that inherited qualities of body tissues predispose some families to joint disease at an earlier age and in more severe forms.

In support of this theory of an inherited susceptibility are studies that show rheumatoid arthritis to be four or five times more frequent in relatives of arthritics than in the general populace. Other scientists argue that this may be a matter of environment, and as findings in support of this they cite the fact that the disease occurs more often among husbands and wives of arthritics than among married couples in general. Also, in studies of identical twins, the disease is often found in one twin and not the other, which, as one scientist states, proves that no simple genetic hypothesis can explain rheumatoid arthritis. Heredity has been ruled out as a definite cause, but is still considered a contributing factor. In other words, no one believes that a person gets arthritis solely because of his genetic make-up, but many believe that genetic factors do make an individual more susceptible to the disease.

A possible dietary role is considered in the study of the causes of any disease. The history of the Maoris of New Zealand reveals they were relatively free from all arthritis except the senile type, until they deviated from their own natural, simple diet, and began eating more processed foods. In America, however, dietary beliefs, whims, and absurdities in connection with rheumatoid arthritis have flourished like weeds and have been just as difficult to uproot. Many of them still flourish in spite of liberal powderings of scientific sanity. Almost every dietetic extreme has had its adherents—high protein, no protein, fruit and vegetable juices, nothing but rice, raw foods, low calcium—to say nothing of the various vitamin crazes, a subject upon which the general public finds it easy to go wild, sometimes abetted by ill-advised statements by scientists, who sometimes get careless about having proofs at hand. One statement in a report in the *Journal of the American Medical Association,* "No particular food item or vitamin has been found to be either beneficial or detrimental in rheumatoid arthritis," should smother all this dietary enthusiasm.

An ambitious individual who approached the Arthritis Foundation with the request "I'd like some funds to help me discover the cause of arthritis" would be dismissed as a dreamer, if not actually taken to be de-mented. The cause of arthritis does not exist as a pre-cious jewel to be unearthed by some lucky prospector. It is more like a jigsaw puzzle, in a multitude of pieces. Probably we have most of the pieces now, perhaps even all of them. What researchers are doing is looking for possible missing pieces and for inspiration in how to fit them all together.

Thus the immediate objectives of arthritis research are apt to be things the general public has never heard of. Often they involve the study of the most minuscule particles recognizable by any known laboratory tech-niques—lysosomes, for example. These have been known for some time, but their characteristics continue to attract scientific scrutiny. It has been stated that the chief function of one class of white blood cells is to engulf and destroy harmful substances. As one au-thority puts it, they are the garbage disposal system of the body. These cells are the polymorphonuclear leuco-cytes, a name which means "white cells with variously shaped nuclei." The lysosomes constitute the mech-anism by which these leucocytes destroy the debris and any other foreign matter they engulf. (The word "lyso-some" means "dissolving body.") These lysosomes are minute sacs, about a hundred to each leucocyte, filled with enzymes which disintegrate the foreign matter.

All this is only background data, accumulated in numerous research studies over a period of years. The tie-in with arthritis has occurred much more recently, when it began to be suspected that these lysosomal enzymes sometimes engage in an aberrant activity that is destructive to body tissues, namely those of the joints. Corroboration or disproof of this suspicion has been the subject of other research projects.

One study done recently in England corroborates

the implication of these enzymes in rheumatic disease without question. The crucial part of this study was the development of an antiserum to the enzymes, which has been demonstrated to cause a significant reduction in the breakdown of cartilage in diseased joints. So far, so good, but what can we do about it? Nothing, at present, except hope that we may be another step nearer the goal. True, we could now stop the joint disintegration caused by these enzymes by giving patients the antiserum, but not without entirely knocking out the enzyme action that safeguards the body. Tampering with the natural protective mechanisms of the body is a risky business, to be undertaken with great caution if at all.

Although this antiserum, which is capable of neutralizing the lysosomal enzymes, is of no known therapeutic value at present, its proven existence is an important step forward in arthritis research. We seem to have come to an impasse in this direction; it is necessary that we choose another course. One favored by recent researchers is directed toward the question of what causes these useful lysosomal enzymes to act in this unreasonable manner at times; to destroy tissues in their own host.

The seeking of this answer thus becomes the nucleus of another, entirely different, research project, which may well supply the most crucial parts of the puzzle. Two possible initiating circumstances are considered. First, that something happens in the immediate environment of the lysosome-bearing white cells to give them a wrong signal, to make tissues of the joint appear to be foreign matter and therefore marked for destruction. Second, that something has been introduced into the body fluids that weakens the walls of the lysosomal sacs so that they rupture too easily, thus recklessly freeing the enzymes of disintegration in the wrong places.

The biggest boost to arthritis research in many years came from the discovery of cortisone, and one of the contributions of cortisone was the demonstration of its impact on the lysosomal sacs. It definitely toughens them, thus diminishing to a remarkable degree the havoc wrought by enzymes permitted to run wild in arthritic joints. This explains in part, perhaps altogether, the relief experienced by arthritics from the administration of cortisone, and is some justification for the early optimistic belief that a long-sought cure was found. However, there are pitfalls and hazards in its use as a treatment (discussed in Chapter 13.)

Faced with these dead ends, the researcher must veer in another direction, which leads him most often to the old, old problem which has come to be the focusing point for all arthritis research—the search for the obscure triggering device, the tinder that sets off the explosion into rheumatoid arthritis. After explorations in all other directions possible to be imagined, researchers return continually to the thought of an infective agent of some kind. It can hardly be an ordinary bacterium, or it would have been identified long ago. The culprit may be a particularly elusive virus, a bacterial variant, or some other little known infective agent such as a mycoplasma.

The research projects alluded to here are a mere sampling of the multitude of studies being pursued. There is a large amount of work being done in the field of drugs, also; seeking greater relief for the millions of sufferers already afflicted, until that hoped-for day when we have a cure. When all the puzzle pieces are fitted into their proper places, the final one will be "Breakthrough" in publicity parlance. But IT would not have been possible without all this supportive work in the background.

In the past twenty-five years the number of research centers studying arthritis has increased from about twelve to more than a hundred. In this same period, the number of universities in the United States offering studies for the training of scientists in arthritis research has increased from five or six to about forty.

From this greater concentration of interest, many new research methods and facilities have emerged. Better laboratory equipment includes improved electron microscopes, ultracentrifuges, column chromatographs, electrophoresis apparatus, tissue culture equipment.

The establishment of NIAMD (the National Institute of Arthritis and Metabolic Diseases) in 1950 was a powerful impetus to research, and cortisone, discovered in 1949, was a powerful impetus to NIAMD. The importance of the discovery of cortisone has already been mentioned, but deserves repeating. Dr. Roger L. Black of the National Institutes of Health, says, "Few clinical discoveries in the history of medicine have had such a profound influence on medical research . . . as has the observation that cortisone can reverse the inflammatory changes of rheumatoid arthritis." This discovery put some hope into the fight against arthritis, which was what it needed to keep it from dying out altogether.

These random details are of little practical use to the arthritis sufferer, but they do afford him a kind of psychological benefit. The victims of all chronic diseases have need of a psychological boost at times, and arthritics are no exception. A simple statement of the facts and figures connected with arthritis research in the past few years offers vast encouragement, without any elaboration or commentary. This hope, moreover, is no ephemeral dream; it is documented.

That the fight against arthritis has now been rejuvenated is an understatement. The rather awesome truth is that for the first time in history man's oldest disease has a purposeful and well-armored campaign mounted against it. The weaponry is scientific expertise, but the ammunition is money. The millions of arthritis sufferers in this country can enlist actively in their own campaign by striving to see that the ammunition does not run short in supply. One single concerted move on their part could accomplish wonders in this direction—and that is to divert to research what they are now spending on quack cures, and to preach this same gospel to all their friends.

IO

Possible Nonphysical
Causes of Arthritis

It has taken a long time, but "psychosomatic" factors have come to be recognized as causes of a great many ills, notably of the digestive system. A child who routinely complains of stomachache before school but at no other time is not apt to be suspected of organic stomach disease. Getting an ulcer has often come to be the price for accomplishment in the business world. No one can deny that psychological factors operate in obesity. A patient once told me that when they remodeled their house, a job that met with many setbacks, she gained thirty pounds in that one summer.

Hindsight being the perspicacious mental faculty that it is, it is difficult for us to understand why the supreme authority of the brain as the controlling mechanism of the entire body, in disease as well as in health, should ever have been questioned. How could a crossing of wires, a tangle of circuits, blockage of a channel in this all-important control center fail to cause some kind of physical malfunction?

Since the beginnings of man we have had evidence of the physical effects of emotions. With the exception of foreign irritants in the eye, the sole cause of tears is emotional—something for the hard-core scientists to swallow. Think of it! Just by feeling badly, those little lachrymal glands can be made to squeeze out such an excess of their watery secretion that it runs out over the cheeks and down through the nose! Other somewhat less dramatic physical responses to emotions have been in existence since the beginnings of man's memory— the flushing of embarrassment, the pallor of fear.

Hindsight makes us wonder why these facts did not point the way sooner to a search for other possible similar happenings. The reason was probably their universality. Familiarity smothers wonder. It is only the rare thinker whose mind is piqued by things he has seen all his life. So it has been a slow, step-by-step process to demonstrate how messages from the control tower direct everything that happens inside the body. What can be seen with the naked eye is the easy part. No controversy there—this nerve goes to this muscle. See it? But emotions are something else. No one has ever followed the path of an emotion along a nerve trunk. No one has ever seen fear, fright, worry, despair. Instead, we see only the cause-and-effect sequence, and much of this is conjectural until we have the statistical support of a great number of similar cases. Even then we do not have proof in the same class with an X-ray picture, a positive reaction in the laboratory, a slide under a microscope.

One of the earliest collections of these cause-and-effect sequences was Pavlov's famous study of the effects of mental stimuli on the digestive system of dogs. It was demonstrated that the sight and smell of food (and later, only the ringing of a bell) could cause an increased secretion of gastric juices and a drooling of saliva. This "Pavlovian" effect has been so solidly established that it has become an idiom of our speech.

The digestive tract makes a good example to cite because of the variety of its points of psychosomatic vulnerability, but there is no reason to believe that any systems are immune. Headache and backache are two of the most common complaints the physician hears. In a great many of these, no organic explanation can be found, and so they are assumed to be of emotional origin. A prolonged tightening of muscles anywhere is an unpleasant sensation, varying from an ache to intense pain. (As mentioned previously, part of the pain of arthritis comes from the contraction of muscles about an inflamed joint.) A muscle is *only* capable of contraction. When it is stimulated or irritated, it simply does its thing, the kind of distress caused by muscle contraction can happen anywhere that there are muscles. The urinary bladder is one such place.

A woman patient came to see me once before starting on a car trip. She said she loved traveling except for one thing: "I always get cystitis [or a bladder infection] the day I start, and it lasts all through the trip. I never have had it at any other time except once, and that was years ago. They found a lot of pus in my urine then, but never at any time since. But I feel just like I did then. I keep getting more and more miserable until we come to the next rest-room stop. Then it is the same thing all over again. It spoils the trip for me and for everyone with me."

Her own diagnosis of cystitis was an erroneous one,

97

as any physician would have suspected from her story. The timing of her symptoms was too pat. Cystitis might synchronize itself with the beginning and end of a trip *once,* but its happening time after time was too much to believe. Having determined that her urine was normal, the logical remaining assumption was that her symptoms were caused by tension of the muscles in her bladder walls. One could surmise that this was brought about in one of two psychological ways. A defeatist attitude would have made her think, "Now that I'm going on a trip, I just *know* my cystitis is going to start up again." Or a too determined antagonism to her problem, "I'm not going to the toilet at every rest stop! I'm not going to let myself!" Either attitude provoked an abnormal mental concentration on her bladder.

I did not go into the psychological aspects of her problem with her. She was already packed for her trip, and the trouble with any kind of psychological adjustment is that it takes time. A mild muscle relaxant is quicker, and it worked. I haven't seen her lately, and do not know how she has fared on recent car trips. What I hope is that having had her bladder eased into the background for this one trip, the excitements and enjoyments of travel have permanently taken precedence in her mind over her bladder.

Other questions follow in logical sequence. Since emotions can do this to the bladder, what else can they do? Are the effects of emotions always as benign as this? Isn't it likely that there are harmful effects, as well as good ones? Now we are in the realm of disease, whether or not we set out for that specific destination. Evidence piles up to inculpate emotional factors in almost everything bad that ever happens to the digestive tract—stomachache, nausea and vomiting, stomach and duodenal ulcer, diarrhea, colitis, ileitis, esophagitis —and somewhere along the way, several of these may have picked up arthritis as a fellow-traveler.

Some possible psychological backgrounds of arthritis seem to cry out for notice, as in the case of the woman who became severely arthritic shortly after the death of her husband. Another case might appear to offer a mute reproach to the physician for not having sensed psychological factors years sooner, as in the case of the woman with arthritis of long standing who got well when her husband died!

The human back has been a source of trouble ever since man stopped getting about on all fours and attempted to hold himself more or less erect. His body design was predicated upon four-legged support instead of two. In adopting this more prideful stance, he was asking for trouble. He got it; and is still having it.

Throughout the centuries much symbolism has come to be attached to the spine. A man "without backbone" is a weak creature. A bent back signifies humility, or the weight of heavy burdens. An "upright man" is a figure of nobility of character. "Stiff-necked" means determination to the point of stubbornness. A "pain in the neck" is suffering in a touchy spot. "Sticking out his neck" implies vulnerability.

As an introduction to his monograph on the psychosomatic aspects of arthritis, psychiatrist Emanuel Miller uses this paragraph from Herman Melville's *Moby Dick:* "I believe that much of a man's character will be found betokened in his backbone. I would rather feel your spine than your skull. Whoever you are. A thin joist of a spine never did uphold a full and noble soul. I rejoice in my spine as in the fine audacious staff of that flag which I fling half out to the world."

. Low-back pain is such a common physical complaint that a possible psychological connection lurks in the background of the mind of even the most hard-core physical scientist. Quoting Emanuel Miller again, "Back pains are frequently found . . . in persons with hysterical withdrawal from stress, sometimes near the frontiers of malingering." And again, in connection with a series of reported cases, "A frequent feature was the 'on guard' attitude." The author held the view that such subjects were in a constant state of readiness yet unable to take action, so that a muscle-bound state supervened and the posture of offense-defense was held, with resulting tension and pain. An arthritic with a background of psychological training corroborates this with a statement about herself: "My own muscular tension, which once in a while seems to lead to a touch of arthritis, derives from being poised between fight and flight—held-back rage and the fear of expressing it. I see this frequently in arthritic people." Psychoanalysts have considered that low-back pain in both sexes is sometimes the result of guilt feelings about masturbation.

A California group, Drs. Alfred A. Amkraut, George F. Solomon, and Helen C. Kraemer, have provided the psychological theory with a laboratory backing by an experiment on rats. According to the scientific report, a group of these animals were subjected to "conditions of stress." What they did was to torment the daylights out of these creatures for a period of a week, keeping them in constant unease by overcrowding in their pens, with no opportunity to relax or rest. Thus dreaming up a situation that was for each comparable to a man's getting out of the office late, standing in a crowded subway, having a fight with his wife after getting home, followed by no appetite for dinner but eating anyway, then having indigestion all night and being unable to sleep.

Scientists know how to induce arthritis in laboratory animals, and this was the crux of the whole experiment. And wouldn't you know it! The rats that had been subjected to the stress got this artificially induced arthritis more promptly and severely, and in a greater number of joints, than those in the control group.

Perfectionists may argue that there is a lot of difference between rats and humans, that what is true of one species may not be true of another. But it seems downright logical that a disruption of the smoothness of the mental processes of any form of life that has anything that passes for a mind could cause disharmony in any part of the organism. What sort of controlling machine would the mind have to be, not to be affected by interference?

A description of any disease takes note of its incidence according to sex. This done, the next step of many "authorities" is to lump in with whichever sexual preponderance is established all the traditional adjectives descriptive of that sex, however archaic and lacking in scientific integrity they may be. Thus rheumatoid arthritis, preponderantly a disease of women, becomes automatically also a disease of the emotionally unstable, of people "especially susceptible and sensitive to environmental conditions, of those accustomed to cyclic physiologic changes and therefore more under the influence of phases of the moon and deeply affected by supernatural phenomena and spiritual beliefs." All of this has been written about the female psyche, and

101

most of it I relegate to the same scrap heap that contains the old notion that gout tends to afflict those of superior intelligence.

Psychic factors may be said to have an effect on every disease, and rheumatoid arthritis is certainly no exception. The very circumstance of indisposition, with its accompanying distress and malfunctioning of various parts, must necessarily provoke some kind of psychological response, coping mechanisms that vary with individual personalities. To prove that a disease is caused by emotional stress alone, becomes a more difficult matter, but not impossible to consider. Some patients have dated the onset of their illness from some shattering emotional experience such as family griefs or economic crises. Few scientists, give credence to these psychic shocks as the primal causes of the disease, however, considering it far more likely that the ingredients were all laid, awaiting only a spark which may be psychic or otherwise, to start the smoldering process of destruction characteristic of this disease.

Some scientists have tried to read common personality traits into victims of rheumatoid arthritis, finding in these people a greater than average proportion of depression, hostility, and resentment. One rheumatologist has said that he considers these patients typically passive, resigned, and long-suffering. The gigantic flaw in all this reasoning is that the studies have been made on people after they have become victims of the disease, not before. Which of us, crippled and suffering, would not develop periods of depression, hostility, and resentment after a time? Some arthritic sufferers have killed themselves because of their prolonged pain and hopelessness. And how could anyone who has endured

years of this disease appear other than pa
signed, long-suffering?

So many personality traits have been reported ~
"typical" of the premorbid arthritic temperament that
if one tried to avoid arthritis by subduing all of them,
he would have to cancel out his personality altogether
and become a robot. I do not wish to impugn the validity of any of these studies or to intimate that they are
without value. Their value increases as they are repeated by other groups in other places, under varying
circumstances. The inevitable results of such labors will
be to sift out the nuggets of truth.

Among the adjectives that have been claimed to
describe the arthritic personality are shy, rigid, moralis-
tic, inhibited, self-conscious, conforming, self-sacrific-
ing, masochistic, perfectionistic. Schizophrenic is on
the list of some observers, who claim to have found
similarities between rheumatoid arthritics and schiz-
ophrenics. If these observers are correct, the fact that
it is most unusual for the two diseases to occur in the
same person would suggest that some of these individuals eventually come to a point at which, however unwit-
tingly, they make a choice between arthritis and schizophrenia.

There must be some connection or some kind of
relationship, between what we call rheumatoid arthritis and what we call schizophrenia, because of the
demonstrated fact that the incidence of arthritis in hospitalized psychotics, who are preponderantly schizo-
phrenics, is significantly less than in the population as
a whole. Dr. D. Gregg published a paper in the *American Journal of Psychiatry* on the paucity of arthritis
among psychotic cases, in which he states that only

103

twenty cases of arthritis were reported in more than fifteen thousand hospitalized psychotics. Allusion has been made in previous chapters to the poorly defined boundaries of rheumatoid arthritis. Trying to correlate this disease with schizophrenia (which psychiatrist R. D. Laing says has no definition at all and may not even exist as an entity) seems a more erratic journey into uncharted space than a discussion which is trying to remain rooted on solid scientific ground.

Any kind of scientist feels himself out on a limb, naked to the scorn of exacting colleagues, unless he can clothe his beliefs in some kind of explanatory garment, however flimsy. So we listen willingly to any theories that sound logical.

One of these has to do with the body's natural immune protective mechanisms, which have a well-proven status. Normally the body has the power to throw out defenses, even attacking forces, against a great many ills that threaten it. Among these are the armies of white cells produced to combat infection; antibodies against specific diseases; injection of extra adrenaline into the blood stream to speed up reaction in time of danger. It seems logical to assume that there are many more that we do not know about. A suggestion of the theorists is that when everything in the body is in normal working order, something, probably one of the endocrine glands, issues an internal prescription for some kind of protective balm to the joints. When anything disrupts the communication system, the order does not get through, and the joints are left vulnerable.

This disrupting factor may well be an emotional one—grief, anger, anxiety, worry, disappointment, discouragement, depression. While these emotions are the common lot of us all, history shows that the damaging

104

effects of such torturings vary almost endlessly among individuals. Some people are only stimulated, others destroyed, and in between these extremes are those whose defense forces are panicked, leaving the victory to whatever enemy is nearest at hand—ulcer, colitis, hypertension, psychosis, or arthritis. Knowledge of these possibilities is a way of being forearmed.

The causes of emotional stress depend upon the underlying personality of the individual and are thus also endlessly varied. Things that tear one person to pieces may leave another comparatively passive. Is there a "rheumatoid personality," and if so, to what extent can one change his personality in an effort to prevent the ravages of arthritic disease? Explorations of this subject enable the individual to build up more effective defenses than he might otherwise. There is no better psychological armor than an understanding of oneself. Trying to draw a picture of the emotional composite most vulnerable to arthritis, however, is a difficult task. A doctor can record with much greater ease and accuracy his findings on a sick patient than he can postulate upon the findings probably present before the patient got sick. This pretty well sums up the difficulties inherent in trying to establish the typical rheumatoid personality (if such a thing exists), but does not deter attempts to describe it.

Not that I believe the psychological causes of disease are mysterious forces beyond the realm of human understanding, without provable scientific integrity. I believe that anything that happens has a *potentially* provable modus operandi, including things called miracles and supernatural happenings, and that the only difference is that some are known and some are unknown.

Loath to accept anything on faith, scientists continue to strive for laboratory proof. Being a scientist of sorts myself, I heartily approve. (I differ from many of them only in my belief that sometimes it is well to act on faith and prove at leisure.) It seems sensible to give these psychological factors the benefit of the doubt, put them on the list of undesirables to be avoided. Why wait to *prove* that they can cause arthritis when some of them (notably stress) are known to be malign factors in other diseases? "Don't get your bowels in an uproar" is recognized as a valid warning against stressful upsets. A similarly pertinent piece of advice might well be, "When you're mad at the boss, don't crunch it out in your joints."

II

Psychological Effects

No disease is solely physical in its harassment. Whatever tortures the flesh, the mind must also record, analyze, and come to grips with in some manner. An acute
illness is apt to require only minor mental adjustments.
Once past the initial shock and dismay, one can usually
cross any chasm of suffering with some equanimity,
seeing hope shining brightly on the other side. Chronic
illness, however, may require mental adjustments of a
more varied and complicated nature. Being committed
to a path of travail with no end in sight makes a gloomy
journey for anyone.

As is to be expected, patients with a terminal illness, those for whom the certain end is death, suffer the
greatest mental strain of all. For many of these, reality
is completely unendurable at first, and they must re-
treat across its borders for a time and find a protective
refuge among the shadows of psychosis, where realities

may be dimmed or even disappear. Then, after a period of recuperation from mental shock, they are often able to come back and face the ravaging truth.

Patients with arthritis find a spot between these possibilities. While the onset may be acute, the course is chronic to the nth degree. Its chronicity, however, seldom contributes to a fatal termination, and the solacing hope of intermission is always present. Since mental attitudes depend primarily upon the psychological make-up of the individuals, it would probably be possible to predict the effects of arthritis upon many people, if one cared to saddle himself with such a research study and had the patience to await the final verdict of time. However, no matter how well he thought he knew his subjects or how carefully he did his psychological testings, no such researcher could achieve complete accuracy. There are hidden strengths and weaknesses in everyone, unknown to even the subjects themselves—traits that require some cataclysmic event to disgorge. Sometimes an illness is such an event, and often arthritis is such an illness, with its unpredictability, its sadistic variety of torturings and its lifelong chronicity. Such an affliction can dredge up unsuspected stores of determination, endurance, hostility, philosophical searchings, resentment, belligerent stimulations, introspection, self-pity. Or, it can crush its victim to an acquiescent inertia, resigned to being a dependent and helpless clod.

With all this variety of psychological findings, it becomes no easy task to determine which of these are predominant; which combine to make a typical picture of an arthritic. My own opinion is that no such "typical" picture exists at the present time. But in all fairness to the researchers, one should examine the findings and conclusions of all widely held interpretations.

Psychiatrist Dermot J. Ward, of Dublin, has reported a group of studies done in that city. These studies used four groups of people—those with early rheumatoid arthritis, chronic rheumatoid arthritics, neurotic patients, and supposedly normal controls. Their findings suggested that people with rheumatoid arthritis differ significantly in personality from normal and from neurotic people, that these differences are accentuated with the chronicity of the rheumatoid process, and that the differences develop as a result of the arthritis. Significantly, this last conclusion takes no note of a premorbid personality, but considers the findings a result of the disease.

One very interesting and unexpected finding of this same research was that the neuroticism score of the early rheumatoids was slightly lower than that of the normals, and the neuroticism score of the patients with chronic rheumatoid arthritis was consistently and significantly lower than that of the normals! Furthermore, it seemed evident that this improvement in the neuroticism scores of the arthritics had occurred after the onset of the disease! At last, it seems there is something good to say about arthritis! In the opinion of these researchers, a substitution occurs in these cases to some degree; an exchange of physical symptoms for the neurotic ones. Thus the individual's health equation would not be a simple "Present morbid state = premorbid state + arthritis," but "Present morbid state = premorbid state + arthritis − x number of neurotic symptoms." In other words, there is a subtraction as well as an addition of pathological symptoms, making the benignity or malignity of the equation dependent upon the severity of the arthritis and the value of x.

An English physician, Henry J. Wyatt, has written an excellent analysis of the factors that bear on the psychological effects of arthritis. Primarily, race and culture are to be considered, since such reactions vary widely among different peoples. In some primitive societies, afflictions may be terrifying beyond the actual suffering involved, being considered a supernatural visitation, perhaps retribution for past misdeeds.

Age correlated with the time of onset of the disease, may be an important factor. When juvenile rheumatoid arthritis comes on in the early months or years of childhood, the effect is less shattering to the morale than when such a crippling disease begins later in life, as the child adjusts from the beginning to its hampered state, knowing no other kind of existence.

Much, perhaps too much, has been said about the role of sex in the psychological effects of arthritis, dumping into the discussion all the attributes of the female sex, real and visionary, since rheumatoid arthritis is predominantly a disease of women.

I shall ignore all these debatable aspects of the feminine psyche, and mention just one wounding effect of arthritis upon mature women that I know to be valid and universal. The onset of arthritis seldom fails to be a dismal warning that a woman is aging. And whatever ameliorations Women's Lib may be able to effect in the future, aging is still much more disastrous to a woman than to a man. A woman with arthritis has no need to look in the mirror to see that this process has set in. She has a constant, nagging awareness that cannot be ignored, from the time she wakens in the morning and finds she cannot roll out of bed with her former agility.

110

"The first gray hairs and wrinkles in the skin are gentle hints that you are getting older," one woman told me, "but nothing gives you the message with a greater jolt than finding, all of a sudden, that you have to limp."

Suicides among men have been attributed to the savage and unrelenting pain of severe arthritis. There seems to me a possibility that arthritis has been a factor quite frequently in suicides among women, who have found unendurable the loss of youth and beauty. Women with great natural beauty possess an irreplaceable asset. No one else can know the psychological trauma suffered in its loss; for some it is too great to bear. What richer target for the sadism of arthritis? And what a varied assortment of reminders to choose from! The shoulders becoming stooped, there are distortions of once lovely hands by enlarged joints and ugly bumps. Shutting the eyes doesn't help. There is no place to hide from it. The aching and the stiffness can be felt just as well in the dark. Whatever depression causes an attractive woman to take her own life, arthritis could very well be a part of it.

Steadfast and firmly held religious beliefs are a source of great strength to many who can find no ease from grief and suffering among the practicalities of living. Unable to see surcease in the hard facts about them, they can close their eyes and believe in things unseen. In some, this is little more than shallow superstition; in others it is an abiding philosophy of life that permeates their entire being. After long, eroding years, some severely afflicted arthritics come to find their greatest serenity in religion. Among these may be many (perhaps most) who had only a perfunctory religious interest in their earlier years. Seeing physical pleasures lessen and become more and more restricted

111

as the years go by, they cling more and more firmly to religion as something they need never lose. In other words, their religion deepens with their arthritis.

A prime example of this in my records is a woman who has been severely crippled from arthritis for years. She was an ambitious, active, determined woman in her youth, greatly averse to "giving in" to anything. Her attitude toward her arthritis was belligerent, never conciliatory or temporizing. Now almost completely helpless, she has turned to religion as her greatest solace, and keeps as a symbolic expression of her own faith, a poem written by another arthritic, Martha Snell Nicholson. In this poem the author tells how "My Lord, and Pain and I" have come to dwell together in sweet harmony and acquiescence. All of which is an about-face from this patient's previous disposition, and probably from that of most arthritics.

The most clearly evident findings in arthritis are always the physical ones. The secondary effects on the psyche are apt to develop more slowly, and may remain hidden from all but the most painstaking diagnostician. Some of them are always present, however, and some that appear mild may be of serious import. Apathy, for example, may be scarcely recognizable as a pathological symptom. The physician might well welcome this attitude as one easy to deal with—no fuss and bother. But in an intelligent person, an apathetic attitude toward a disease that carries threats of a chronic invalidism may indicate that the patient lacks normal drive and initiative, which worsens his prognosis. Such a patient may not be normally cooperative in treatment, and may lapse into early helplessness.

Dependence may be one of the dismaying results of beginning arthritis. Once established, it becomes as chronic as the primary disease itself. Someone to take care of you, being certified by a doctor as unable to work, bills paid by insurance, family, charity, or other outside help—these are emoluments not easily cast aside. Having become completely dependent, physically, financially, and morally, the way back up on one's own feet is a more difficult climb than most are able to make.

Anxiety, bewilderment, fear, frustration, depression, and impatience are all normal reactions to illness to be expected in some degree. But when any of them, especially depression, become greatly exaggerated, they may develop into pathological symptoms necessary to be dealt with on their own score.

Denial is occasionally the initial reaction to the diagnosis of arthritis. In most of my cases it has risen out of intense fear. The patient has known someone, probably a relative, who has suffered the most devastating crippling effects of the disease, lying inert and completely helpless for months or even years before death. Such a tragic case is fixed in the patient's mind as the classic picture of arthritis, the preponderance of lesser afflictions failing to qualify.

The outstanding example of denial among my cases, however, arose from pride rather than fear. This was a ninety-year-old woman who took great satisfaction (as, indeed, who would not?) in the fact that she had never had any arthritis. If the onset of her aging had been distressful to her, it was now so long ago she had forgotten it. She had ridden over that rocky road to a plateau of pride in her years, enjoying somewhat the same kind of glamour that a beautiful woman has in her prime. Her good health and energy, her mental acuteness, excellent figure and carriage, and agility

113

were remarkable for her years, and commented upon freely by all who knew her. Then one day in the course of a minor acute illness she developed a stiff, swollen, and painful knee. She never asked me what was the matter with her knee, and I never told her, so the dread word never passed between us. The antiarthritic I prescribed for her was very efficient, and to this day, as far as I know, no doctor has ever told her she had arthritis.

Just as the effects of an illness are never solely physical, so are the effects never limited to the patient alone. An illness impinges not only upon those who take care of a patient, but to a varying extent upon those who care about him. Chronic illnesses such as arthritis constitute one of the great burdens of society. Identification and analysis of the effects of arthritis on these secondary sufferers are the basis of numerous studies being pursued at the present time, and there are probably endless approaches to these problems that have not yet been opened.

One group of researchers at the University of Michigan, Dr. Sidney Cobb, Stanislav V. Kasl, John R. P. French, and Guttorm Nörstebö, did an interesting study based on a hunch of Dr. Cobb's. His hypothesis, briefly stated, was that women with rheumatoid arthritis should be married to men with peptic ulcer. Stated thus briefly, and read hastily as I read it first, it sounded like an amazing piece of advice in eugenics. His meaning, of course, was that this state of affairs ought to be true—given certain known psychological characteristics of arthritics and of ulcer patients—and Dr. Cobb and his co-workers set out to prove that it is true in a far greater number of cases than could be set down to coincidence. They believe the explanatory key to be marital hostility, which contributes to rheumatoid ar-

114

thritis in the wife by way of resentment and depression, and to peptic ulcer in the husband by way of unmet needs for emotional support.

Probably no form of arthritis equals the juvenile type in its variety of family-permeating effects. No member of the immediate family is immune to the psychological miasma that surrounds a child with a chronic, crippling illness, and the worry and concern often spread to relatives in distant places, especially grandparents. In fact, I wonder sometimes if the emotional strain on grandparents is not even greater. The parents are occupied, busy in the battle for the child's recovery, or improvement, whichever they dare hope for, and fighting for something gives a certain emotional release of its own. The grandparents, on the other hand, can do little but worry and hope and pray.

The burdens imposed upon the immediate family by the chronic illness of a child may best be considered in three categories—financial, physical, and emotional. Of these, the major financial concern is usually borne by the father, the other two by the mother. The mother usually has the hygienic and nursing care of the child. She attends to his medications and exercises, if they are a part of his regimen as they are apt to be in arthritis. She watches fearfully and hopefully for signs of improvement or worsening of his illness, often imagining the one or the other where it does not exist, according to the vagaries of her own temperament. In general, she must do all the necessary things for his physical care, and in addition try to keep him from becoming bored, unhappy, and discouraged. She must be on the alert continually for ways to boost his morale; teach, amuse, entertain; temper sympathy, at times, with firmness; expect and insist upon the right amount of cooperation. Who of us has ever done the job perfectly? I should say unequivocally that the mother of a child with a chronic, handicapping illness has the most difficult nursing job in the world.

A mother's initial reaction to such a situation is apt to be that natural human response to anything that seems intolerable, to refuse to believe it. "It can't be true!" "The doctor must be mistaken!" "Let's ask someone else!"

After the bitter acceptance may come a period of guilt, vindictiveness, resentment, acrimony. Both parents may share a feeling of guilt, or each may secretly blame the other for fancied neglect or other culpability. These feelings are apt to be less intense in the father than in the mother, for the simple reason that during the working day the father is away from home. Whatever the rigors of his working life, at least he is in contact with normalcy, away for a time from the emotional and pathological problems—all of which attests to the validity of what I believe to be one of the most important safeguards for the mother's mental stability. She, too, should get away from the house for short intervals, and taking the afflicted child for a walk to the park or the zoo will not suffice. Although there is probably no piece of advice that she will resist more stubbornly, she should have some time away from the child. It may require much argument and persuasion to convince her that leaving her sick child for occasional brief intervals is not a dereliction of duty on her part, but a necessary recuperative adjunct to her own mental strength, from which her entire family, including the sick child, will benefit as much as she does.

Occasionally the mother of such a child has found the duty of care beyond endurance and has left her family or taken her own life. Most cope as best they can, however, with their shortened day-to-day vision. It is only in later years, when they can look back with some perspective, that they see their errors and shortcomings glaring at them. Lack of devotion to the afflicted child is seldom one of these errors. More often there has been a lack of ability to see past the sick child to the needs of the others in the family. Seeing all the needful care and attention heaped upon the one child, the others may come to believe that they hold a lesser place in the mother's affection or even fail to share in it at all. This may come as an anguished realization to the mother in later years. How could she have been so blind, so thoughtless and neglectful, as to fail to recognize their little gropings for more of her time and tenderness?

Catastrophic as such an affliction is to a family, there are a few pitiful benefits that accrue. In spite of their occasional spoutings of rebellion and resentment, children who grow up in such an atmosphere can scarcely fail to learn more about tolerance, helpfulness, and compassion than their contemporaries know. I once overheard a conversation between two little boys in which one of them was expressing curiosity about a crippled member of the family of the other. "She can't walk," explained the boy who was being interrogated. "And don't you laugh, either!" he added with protective belligerence.

117

Part Three

Treatment

12

Prevention

A summary of all the treatments for arthritis (or for any other disease) leaves much to be desired. Whatever their virtues, the entire lot of them is still only second best to the optimum accomplishment—prevention. No matter how brilliant a cure the researchers eventually come up with, nothing beats never having had the disease at all.

Try to prevent something of which we do not know the cause? The concept is not as visionary as it seems at first thought. Paradoxically, more optimism can be infused into a discussion of the *prevention* of arthritis than into any other phase of the battle against it. Let us leave to the scientists the final answer as to whether the cause of arthritis is infectious, hormonal, allergic, autoimmunal, or whatever, and concentrate on some of those secondary or contributory causes which we *do* know about and which almost everyone admits are a part of the picture—and about which we can take some action.

Physical factors that may be contributory to arthritis, such as infection, chilling, joint overuse, have been mentioned previously, and once identified, suggest their own defensive approaches. Stress has an important place in this group also—physical stress being one of the well-recognized causes of joint damage. There is probably no overweight woman seeking treatment for arthritis whose doctor has not urged, even demanded, that she reduce the load her tortured knee joints have to bear.

Practically all the theories presently held about the cause of arthritis take into account a supplementary "triggering" factor without which (even with the primary cause all set to go) the final explosion into this destructive disease might not take place. There is overwhelming evidence that some of these triggers may be psychological and, as such, not demonstrable by laboratory methods and therefore not readily accepted as scientific fact. A passive acceptance of any kind of suffering is not good. Feeling discouraged, brokenhearted, sick about something, is a mental morass one should get out of as quickly as possible. Lying inert, you could get sicker, and in a variety of ways.

The converse is not exactly true, however. Pushing oneself to the limit, day after day, has a wearing effect on the entire body. A good sermon I have just read on this subject is by Roy L. Minich, in his little volume, *Bread for the Journey.* He tells of an explorer in South America who followed such a strenuous regime in his trek through the jungles that one morning his porters failed to appear. His head man explained, "We have traveled far and we have traveled fast; we must now wait for our souls to catch up with our bodies."

Sometimes a change of activity can be more beneficial than a complete rest. I once had a discussion with
a woman writer who had just finished a book and sent
it to her publisher with grave misgivings. It was not a
book they had encouraged her to write, but something
she herself wanted to do anyway. The writing of the
book had been an arduous task, and after the manuscript was in the mail, she decided to take a rest before
starting anything else. "I think that's where I made my
mistake," she told me, and I agreed with her. Her mind
was idling during the ensuing weeks but not resting,
being bombarded constantly by her doubts and anxie-
ties about the fate of the book. She would have done
far better to plunge immediately into her next piece
of writing, and to leave the resting until after the
anxiety-fraught period of waiting was over, however it
should terminate. Sometimes waiting for a blow can be
more damaging than the blow itself. As it was, she made
herself as vulnerable as possible to whatever punishment the fates had in store for her, and in about two
months she had an acute attack of rheumatoid arthritis
which was partially crippling. She had had some arthritic disease before, but nothing like this. By the time
she told me of it, she was back to her usual state of
health, and she herself believed that her emotional
stress had been the cause of this episode of illness.

Treating rheumatoid arthritis is not a matter of
giving the patient a prescription for some pills. The
prescription is usually a part of the treatment, but it
follows other basic considerations. The patient's personality and his living habits are to be considered
primarily. The type of work a patient does has a great
deal to do with what it takes to incapacitate him. It is
coming to be believed more and more strongly that his
temperament is a factor in his having developed the

disease in the first place, and in the progress he makes under treatment.

An intelligent and unusually perceptive woman with severe rheumatoid arthritis explained her own feelings to me: "I know I've got to stop pushing myself so hard, or I'll never get better. But that's easier said than done. I've always been like that. When we were first married, and I was teaching school as well as keeping house, my husband would say to me in the evenings, 'Why don't you sit down and watch TV with me for a while? Let some of the work go.' I couldn't see that I was punishing myself by working. It was what I liked to do; I enjoyed getting things done. I wonder now if I would have been any better off sitting there and watching TV, all the while fretting about the work I was neglecting. Wouldn't that have been just as upsetting to me?"

A difficult question to answer. How does one change one's personality? It is too preposterous a goal to set for oneself. Better to settle for a moderation, as this woman has done. It seems to me that she has done a great deal toward helping herself by her understanding of the personality factors that have been operative in her case, and tempering her drives down to a less demanding level; in other words, she is learning to travel in a lower gear.

Etiologic studies continue to find more and more evidence of the influence of the emotions on both the cause and the progress of disease. Helping patients understand this is a valuable part, in fact, the proper beginning, of treatment. Knowledge that one's ambitions, fears, griefs, worries, carry the threat of ulcer, colitis, hypertension, arthritis, and probably many more bodily punishments is the beginning of wisdom. Not that

serenity can be had for the seeking, but being fore-
warned enables the patient to marshal whatever defenses are available.

Aggression is one of the most important character
traits in motivational psychology and is considered to
be one of the most powerful drives in the human
psyche. One single statistic is enough to establish a connection between aggression and arthritis—the fact that
the incidence of arthritis in penal institutions is significantly lower than in the population at large (no pun
intended). What an inspiration to the devil for sermon-
izing! "Smart people release their aggressive instincts,
and don't get arthritis! Rob and clobber your fellow
man when you feel like it, and stay well!" (Staying out
of prison need not be mentioned.) The obligation all
this lays upon the law-abiding therapist is plain to be
seen. It is to suggest *benign* ways for the release of
aggressive instincts. No specific outlines for such therapy have yet been suggested.

Possibilities seem as varied as personalities themselves. A man of my acquaintance with a very aggressive personality was able to work off his aggressive
drives in a very useful manner throughout a busy
professional life. When he retired, his wife told me that
she worried a great deal about his adapting himself to
a more peaceful existence. She has reported to me
since, from time to time, that he is doing very well. He
is a "morning person," one of those who wake with the
feeling that they could conquer the world and feel ea-
ger to get at it. ("He wakes up chirping," says his wife,
who is decidedly not a morning person herself, and who
finds early morning exuberance little to her liking.) This
man starts releasing his aggressive feelings as soon as
he gets downstairs and picks up the newspaper. His

reading is punctuated by vehement and often explosive verbal commentary. Being a methodical person, he starts with the headlines and goes on through: "Those foreign bastards will take us for everything we've got!" "How come school kids think they can run things?" "Why don't they do something about those hijackers?" "This paper is as biased as hell!" "That Clark Mollenhoff is going to get himself shot! Nobody can keep after crooked politicians and underworld figures the way he does and live a very long life!"

Having finished off the newspaper he often goes to the basement. His wife doesn't know what he does in the basement, but she hears him pounding things. Or, in the summer months, he spends most of his day on the lawn, decapitating the withered blooms from the iris, amputating accessory branches from lilacs and other shrubbery, fighting the crabgrass. "There's never a dull moment for him," his wife says, "and he never seems bored."

Here is one aggressive personality, then, who has never landed in jail, and he has only a minimal amount of arthritis. His way of life would perhaps not suit anyone else. The connotation in this account is that there are oases of content for other personalities, to be had for the seeking, and that the balm of serenity has as beneficial an effect on the entire being as do the therapeutic baths on arthritic human joints, or the warm muck of the swamps on those of the prehistoric reptiles.

Realizing that there are preventive measures we can take to ward off any kind of trouble is a morale booster in itself. It makes arthritis seem a little less inexorable, shows some of the vulnerabilities in the disease itself, strengthens our determination to take a stand against it instead of helplessly accepting defeat. It is a well-known fact that the patient who puts up a good fight and has a strong determination to get well greatly increases his chances for recovery. There are case histories illustrating this tenet that sound miraculous. The scientific sequence of events in such recoveries is not readily explainable, but it seems possible for a similar sequence to occur in recovery from these psychological traumas, just as a period of prostration following a grief or worry or any other emotional bruising is a period of greatest vulnerability to other ills.

A friend of mine gave me an account of some trouble she had with her back many years ago. It lasted over a period of four years, and at times was almost completely disabling. She had such intense muscle contractures that she could not bend her back, and sometimes had to be helped out of bed and into an erect posture; all of which was extremely painful. Her physicians told her that they could find no evidence of arthritis or of any other organic trouble. She was having very worrisome psychological problems at the time, she told me, but she is now completely well. She still has no evidence of arthritis, and her back is as limber as anyone's. The source of her psychological distress, however, did not disappear. What, then, "cured" her?

Studying her problem from the vantage point of time, I feel convinced that she did most of it herself. True, she had excellent supportive therapy from both her physicians, and perhaps she could not have done it without their help. Attentive and sympathetic, they worked assiduously to relieve her localized symptoms. Most important of all, she liked and trusted them, both as people and as physicians. When they assured her there was "nothing wrong" organically, she believed them implicitly, and this knowledge gave her a firm foundation from which to begin recuperation.

She is a highly intelligent woman with a stable

personality, unselfish, and attentive to the needs of her family. At that time she had a husband and two children. These were the hard facts that faced her: there was nothing wrong with her that she couldn't get over; her family needed her; she *had* to get well. She must have searched her mind frantically for the "coping devices" that all of us need at times to see us through trouble. She did tell me of one small enlightening incident. At Christmastime in one of her bad years she could not straighten her back; she had to walk all hunched over and pulled to one side. She felt hardly able to be up, but marring her family's Christmas was unthinkable to her. So she made the day a festive one, getting about in her crippled posture and telling the children, "This is old Mrs. Claus, come to help out Santa this year."

It has pleased me very much to report this case history, as a possible help and inspiration to others. It serves as a good example of what Dr. Karl Menninger means when he says that we all have some coping devices to help us through psychological troubles, and that we should always try to seek them out. It also bolsters my opinion that much can often be accomplished by self-help in psychiatric therapy.

If asked whether I think arthritics get a sufficient amount of psychological attention, I should have to say no. Case records of arthritics are dotted with occurrences that point to unrecognized psychological factors that influenced the earlier stages of the disease. One example is that of a man badly crippled for years with arthritis, confined to a wheelchair, and almost helpless. After the death of his devoted wife, he attained a much greater degree of self-sufficiency.

This is by no means an uncommon happening in

family circles that include a badly handicapped member. What looks like neglect of a handicapped person is sometimes the best kind of therapy. But its apparent cruelty is a strong deterrent to its voluntary use, and its achievement usually requires firm and persistent encouragement on the part of someone outside the family from whom they are willing to accept direction—most commonly the family physician. To watch a loved one straining to do some simple thing with his crippled hands and refrain from doing it for him is almost impossible. In most instances it cannot be done without keeping the idea of benefit uppermost in one's mind. One of the clear duties of the doctor in management of his arthritis cases is a psychological supervision. Few of us fulfill this obligation completely. I must confess to a personal as well as a professional laxness in this respect. Only in later years did I realize that when I resumed the practice of medicine during the war, leaving my handicapped daughter to the less strict supervision of others during the day, she made the greatest improvement of any era in her entire life!

There is no more potent elixir for the human spirit than to see something beautiful or useful take form as a result of one's own creative efforts. Nothing puts quite the same satisfaction into that terrible void of uselessness. I know a man who, during convalescence from frequent illnesses, found he had an unusual talent for exquisite needlepoint. His work has been displayed widely, and art critics have placed a high value on many of his canvases.

Renoir was a victim of partially crippling arthritis, but he painted with brushes extended on rods. Every year we buy Christmas cards from the Handicapped Artists group, who have to work with similar mechanical aids. My daughter Virginia corresponds with a boy who taps out letters on his electric typewriter with a rod attached to a band around his forehead. Christy Brown, of Dublin, who has written several books that have brought him literary acclaim, does his typing with a stick attached to his big toe. A philologist with hands badly crippled by arthritis, compiled a dictionary in two oriental languages, the letters of which required a considerable dexterity.

Emanuel Miller suggests that the apparent fortitude often displayed by women with rheumatoid arthritis may in reality be an expression of their repressed feelings of rebellion against the "feminine" role they are expected to play in life, denying them the creative outlets they are secretly yearning for. Perhaps this explains why more women than men suffer from rheumatoid arthritis. It will be interesting to note whether the Women's Liberation Movement will alter these statistics.

Nurses and social workers can establish a kind of rapport with a patient that is not duplicated in any other relationship. Lying helpless, the subject of tender, solicitous care, is an experience most patients have not had since infancy, and it cannot fail to have a psychological impact. Whether this is all good or not depends upon whether the patient is able to emerge from his sheltered hiding place within a reasonable interval and face his adult problems and duties again. It is to be hoped that he will be, and that in this respite from his usual cares he will have built up some new sources of enduring psychological strength. Many patients have treasured and cultivated this new friendship with a nurse for the rest of their lives.

The home environment may be the source of an

endless variety of psychological problems for the arthritic. I shall mention sex in passing. Thinking of something new to say on that subject is difficult at best, and I really do believe that there are quite a few other things that human beings think about and worry about sometimes. Among them are concerns about financial income, levels of security, spending habits of the family, job uncertainties, planning for the future, status in the community, frustrations to ambition, family interrelationships. The list could go on and on.

Sometimes I get to thinking that every figure in the limelight of fame, seemingly at the pinnacle of success, is really a frustrated something else. (So, of course, are a great many of us common folk.) A politician who wanted to be an actor, but who was pressured into something more orthodox, compensates by finding his own substitute stage. I can think of a comedian who wanted to be an orchestra leader; an authority on economics who wanted to be a novelist—and tried, once; the drama critic who wanted to be a playwright; the countless housewives who want to write poetry, and do it in spite of everything. More power to all of them! They have found solutions to their own problems.

A discussion of psychological therapy for arthritics at the sub-psychiatrist level does not tell the whole story, of course. Many arthritics do need professional psychological treatment. The doctor in charge tries to keep this in mind and is alert to expressions from patients that suggest deeply buried traumas, such as "What have I done to deserve this?" implying considerations of guilt. A continuing or deepening depression also rings an alarm bell for him.

They are the ones who need help.

13

Drugs and Quack Remedies

It is only logical that to fix something one should know what is wrong, and, if possible, how it happened. This is true in both worlds, organic and inorganic. As long as the cause of a disease remains unknown, it provides a constant challenge, a riddle that *must* be solved before a course of effective treatment can be set. This undying determination is nowhere more evident than in rheumatology, where there is no thought of giving up the battle.

Lacking the knowledge of what causes arthritis, we must do the next best thing, which is to combat the ill effects. In arthritis, this means to relieve the distress, restore function as far as possible, correct deformities that have occurred. The most urgent necessity, as a rule, is the relief of pain, and this usually calls for the use of drugs. Before prescribing these specifics, however, the doctor will wish to know the type of arthritis

133 — 137

he is dealing with. Drugs are used in some kinds of arthritis that would be useless or even hazardous in others.

The treatment of gout is an outstanding example. The use of aspirin, that universal pain reliever in all other kinds of arthritis, is restricted in gout, its use being advised only under the direction of a physician. On the other hand, colchicine which was discussed earlier, is used for gout but for no other kind of arthritis, except in cases in which the diagnosis is in doubt. It is so specific for gout that doctors may use it briefly as a therapeutic test for diagnosis. If an arthritic patient is helped by colchicine, it suggests strongly that the arthritis is the gouty type.

Treatment of arthritis that is secondary to specific known infection, such as gonorrhea, is essentially the treatment of the primary disease. The same is true of the arthritis of rheumatic fever, in which the joints are never the primary concern.

With the exceptions noted in the foregoing paragraphs, the treatment of arthritis in general is not specialized according to types of the disease. It is specialized even more sharply according to individuals. Thus in some types, such as ankylosing spondylitis and systemic lupus erythematosus, no specific treatment is outlined as a general rule. As there is no known cure, the most effective procedures in the arthritic regimen are sought for each case. The statement "no known cure" has a dismal, hopeless sound. To offset it one should always add an equally true statement: "There is no case of arthritis for which something cannot be done."

Since rheumatoid arthritis is the center of the research attention being given to the arthritic diseases, it is natural that rheumatoid arthritis should also be the radiating center for treatment. Most kinds of treatment found effective in this disease have also been found useful in some other kinds of arthritis. Thus what may appear to be favoritism toward rheumatoid arthritis is really a beneficence to the entire group, as the rheumatoid type often acts as a testing ground for them all.

Once the diagnosis of rheumatoid arthritis is made, one of the earliest necessities in treatment is some medication to suppress the inflammatory process as far as possible and to relieve pain. The list of drugs currently available for such purposes is an imposing one, but this is not so desirable as it sounds. It means that no one of them is sure-fire; if it were, there would be no need for alternatives. Thus there would be more optimism in one or two drugs than in a list; drugs such as quinine for malaria, or penicillin for bacterial infections. This fact was well illustrated by an eminent rheumatologist in a lecture he gave to practicing physicians. He made an outline of the drugs used for rheumatoid arthritis, which filled one section of the blackboard. At the close of his lecture he made the dismal observation, "And we don't know how a damned one of them works." Not "how it works," it is true, but that it *does* work in a sufficient number of cases to make each a valuable adjunct to the treatment. The "how" will be better understood when the causes of arthritis are completely unraveled.

Aspirin heads the list of antiarthritic drugs, not only by alphabetical right but because of its universality of use.

Considering all kinds of arthritis, the most commonly used drug is aspirin. In osteoarthritis, it may be the only drug prescribed. Since inflammation is not a factoi here, what is needed is something that will best relieve the aching, stiffness, and soreness of joints that are showing the effects of wear and tear. Probably the only patients treated for any kind of arthritis who have not been given aspirin are those few who are allergic to it. It should not be looked down upon because it is so common; it *is* common precisely because it is one of the most useful drugs we have. It not only relieves pain; it suppresses inflammation also, which explains its value for rheumatioid arthritis as well as for the entire range of systemic infections with fever and aching. But before you watch any more television commercials, order those booklets from the Arthritis Foundation! Then you will be prepared to resist gulping aspirin at the first twinge of pain. A twinge is no indication for aspirin or any other kind of medication. Get the idea out of your head that "treatment" is synonymous with "taking something." Many times it is not. Use the aspirin when you have continuing aches bad enough to be noticeable to you whatever you are doing or to bother your rest at night. Otherwise skip it.

You have already read, in those arthritis booklets, how useful a medication aspirin is, in arthritis as well as in a great many other ills. It is, indeed, "the medicine doctors prescribe." But what the medicine doctors prescribe is acetyl salicylic acid, usually written "ASA, grains V," not "Brand Name" aspirin of the same dosage-size tablets. What's the difference? Nothing that I know of, except the name and the price. Naturally you have to pay a little more for the brand name—think of what the advertising must cost! Most people feel a little safer buying something they have heard of before, something they have seen advertised. If you are one of those, and you doubtless are, go ahead and buy the

136

brand name. Besides, its neat packaging probably appeals to you, too. And there's no harm as long as you have the facts down straight.

The most controversial group of drugs used for arthritis are the corticosteroids. People know them under a variety of names—cortisone, prednisone, prednisolone, dexamethasone, and others. They can be called effective, miraculous, seductive, treacherous, dangerous, sometimes useless, according to experiences with them. It is easy to see, then, why physicians use them with great caution. Some doctors do not prescribe them at all.

One of the painful experiences a doctor may have is to prescribe corticosteroids as a last resort for a patient with severe rheumatoid arthritis who has had no relief from other medications and to have the new medicine give such prompt and marked relief that the patient is ecstatic, thinking, "Now, at last my arthritis is done for. I have some medicine I can depend on." Now comes the difficult part—to have to tell the patient that the prescription cannot be continued over a long period, that it must eventually be stopped, and that there is a chance that the arthritis will be as bad as ever, or even worse, after the medication is stopped. Why prescribe it, then, in the first place? Because sometimes we are lucky. Often the medication can be tapered off gradually over a period of days without any exacerbation of symptoms, and sometimes the patient can be free of symptoms for a long time afterward. In some cases, the doctor's philosophy is that anything is worth a try.

One case which tried my philosophical acumen was that of a woman in her early eighties, whose long-existing rheumatoid arthritis had become worse as she aged. When nothing else worked for her any longer, I prescribed steroids for her, which gave her gratifying relief. Each time I tried to taper off her dosage, however, her joints would flare back to their former inflamed state, with all the former pain and stiffness. I had a serious talk with her, telling her that it was imperative that she get along with much less of this medicine or dire problems might well be in store for her. "But, doctor," she protested, "when I try to do without what I am taking now, I can't get out of bed in the morning." Should I continue the steroids, or permit this elderly woman to become bedfast? I elected to continue the steroids. She lived to her late eighties, and led a fairly active life. She did develop the typical "moon face" as a side effect, but this did not trouble her much, and she suffered no other bad consequences.

Abnormal deposits of fat may occur when patients have taken steroids over a long period. This "moon face" is the most noticeable type of fat deposition that occurs, causing the face to look round and swollen. Other side effects may be skin disorders and abnormal growth of hair. There may be weakening of the bones, making the patient more liable to fractures. Patients with a tendency to stomach or intestinal ulcers are poor risks for steroid therapy. Steroids may cause new ulcers, or reactivate old ones. The symptoms of infections may be masked by steriods, allowing the infections to develop to a serious level before they are recognized.

It was my misfortune, and that of another patient of mine, to have one of the rarer side effects of steroids occur—a mental disturbance. This patient's arthritis improved gratifyingly after only a brief interval of steroid medication, but she developed a depression from which it took her several months to recover. Happily she recovered from her depression, and neither that or her arthritis has recurred. Needless to say, she has not received and will never receive any more steroids.

In spite of all these complaints registered against them, the steroids remain a valuable part of our arsenal against arthritis. Physicians find sometimes that there is nothing that effectively replaces a continued very small dosage of steroids as accessory medication in stubborn cases of rheumatoid arthritis. Also, they may be used locally as injections into affected joints, without any of these systemic side effects.

Researchers are continually looking for medications with a minimum of side effects which are helpful to rheumatoid arthritis sufferers, and they have found some good ones. Phenylbutazone is widely used. The most recent notable one is indomethacin, which has given excellent results in many cases. One thing greatly in its favor is that it may be used over long periods of time with no serious side effects. Injections of gold salts have been used for many years in treatment of rheumatoid arthritis, enthusiasm for them having waxed and waned, with never any unanimity of opinion as to their benefits. They are toxic and must be used with caution. Derivatives of quinine have their proponents for treatment of arthritis in selected cases.

As has been stated, the drug treatment of arthritis is a highly individualized matter. What is beneficence to one patient may be anathema to another. Any doctor who treats arthritis can verify this from his own experience. The first patient for whom I prescribed phenylbutazone told me that her arthritis was better after she took the first tablet. I attributed her enthusiasm to the psychic effect of a new medication, but for her the benefits from it never wore off. Her enthusiasm affected me, too, and I gave it to a number of other patients; many were helped, quite a few were not. On the other hand, when indomethacin came out with glowing reports on its trials at university centers, I gave it to a series of patients with results that supported its reputation. Then another patient to whom I gave it became violently ill after swallowing her first blue-and-white capsule and was in bed for two days with an incapacitating headache. Did the capsule do it? There might have been a question in my mind, but there was none in hers. For her, this first indomethacin capsule was also the last one.

Arthritis is the richest disease field for exploitation by quacks. The facts about it appear to combine in a gigantic invitation to chicanery.

The erratic and unpredictable behavior of the disease itself helps purveyors of quack remedies. Severe one day, better the next; moving from one joint to another; disappearing altogether for a time. Who can blame the hopeful sufferer for thinking, again and again, that he has finally found something that helps? And why count the cost, if the new remedy, however weird and improbable it sounds, can make him well again?

This kind of thinking makes possible the rich harvest being garnered yearly by a multitude of fake arthritis remedies. It has been estimated that there are as many as four hundred such "aids," their number being limited only by the bounds of unscrupulous ingenuity. These include a great variety of electrical devices, lamps whose health-giving rays cannot be demonstrated but need only to be imagined, radioactive pads, massaging apparatus, baths in magic waters. We people in medicine must look to our own shortcomings, because quackery tends to flourish automatically where medicine has failed. Our current endeavors have not yet compensated for the many centuries during which there have seemed to be more important problems to claim our attention. "Why worry about the arthritic? He'll probably outlive us all." Different attitudes now prevail. Apathy has been replaced by persistent and determined efforts by some of the best minds in medical research to dig out the last elusive facts about arthritis that will establish the cause beyond all doubt and point the way to a cure. After this has been done, the promotion of bogus "cures" will gradually shrivel and disappear.

Some of these cures are little more than token offerings to superstition. Carrying a buckeye in the pocket, for example, is about as harmless as anything one can imagine. Copper bracelets are in the same category, unless the patient has paid an exorbitant price for them. I have often put a blood pressure cuff on the arm of a man or woman without commenting on the bracelet at the wrist. I think that in combating quackery a doctor should concentrate on those things that are physically harmful or a financial strain, and there are enough to bear talking about.

A picture that seems to me a composite of all the gullibility and chicanery involved in these schemes is a group of people with crutches and wheelchairs, some of them having traveled long distances, in a series of sessions in which they sit in a worked-out uranium mine, pitifully hopeful that they are absorbing some curative emanations. This underground and underhanded "clinic" has been operating for about twenty years. How can it have survived so long if it does no good? Again, the vagaries of the disease are the explanation, plus the euphoria engendered in patients by a new hope of cure. They feel better for having taken a trip and visiting with other hopefuls, with a mutual exchange and stimulation of enthusiasms, much like the old religious revival meetings. Most of these will testify that they have received some benefit, if questioned at a propitious time, and no one can disprove their allegations.

If a fellow arthritic named Jerry Walsh ever makes a speech in your vicinity, do go to hear him. He has talked to interested groups in many cities, reporting his findings as an "undercover investigator" for the Arthritis Foundation. Probably no one person knows more than he does about these bogus treatments for arthritis. He has traveled all over the country, with the help of crutch and cane, visiting places that advertise arthritis cures and collecting samples of medications and gadgetry. His collection includes over four hundred items, some of which he carries about with him in his "quack bag" to show his audiences. He has also gathered data about the cost of each. There are some designed to milk all financial brackets; one machine costs the patient $800, a more modest one $22.50, with varying prices in between. (The estimated value of this cheaper contraption is three dollars' worth of metal, nothing else.)

Jerry Walsh surveys the whole market of off-color arthritis treatments for you, which will tend to tone down the dazzle of any specific one you may have been directed toward. Listening to him will certainly steer you away from ways of wasting your money.

All of these trickeries, however, are not doing the patients physical harm. They are reprehensible only because they are cheating people. Of greater concern to physicians are the drug mixtures being offered to the public. These are not the seductive but comparatively harmless vitamins-in-alcohol that have made some tonic manufacturers rich. These arthritis "cures" contain potent drugs (among them hormones and the previously mentioned corticosteroids) which are dispensed freely and recklessly, without supervision. Many harmful effects, even some deaths, have been reported from the use of these medications. The most notorious potion, Liefcort, has been banned in this country, but many of our citizens fly to Canada or Mexico to obtain it. One enterprising doctor in Mexico has increased his already flourishing practice by prescribing it as a cure for cancer as well as arthritis.

If paid into the needy coffers of arthritis research, this astronomical amount of money being wasted on quackery every year would bring all these costs closer to a termination. The promotion of this ideal for arthritis-spending must be an educational one, best achieved through publicity for the Arthritis Foundation. All arthritics and their relatives should be aware of the Foundation—the kind of work it does, the help it can offer, the information it has at hand to be had for the asking, its nearest contact points. They should be aware, also, of its need of funds, which it will allocate most advantageously to the ultimate benefit of all.

14

Surgery and Physiotherapy

For the most part surgical treatment of arthritis is an erroneous concept. No surgical procedure has ever cured any kind of arthritis or has ever been performed with that end in mind. In the great majority of cases, surgery is done to repair damage caused by that destructive disease, and in many instances it can restore a miraculous degree of function to areas where it had seemed hopelessly lost. Dr. Andrew Dale of Nashville recently wrote a description of a new procedure of his in peripheral vascular surgery and titled his article, "Salvage of the Extremity." It seems as apt a title as could be found for a number of bone-joint operations also, which restore varying degrees of function to an extremity made useless by the inroads of this disease.

Sometimes, however, the joint deterioration is so severe that complete relief is not possible with normal dosages of any of the pain-relieving drugs, or even with

145

relief of the pain, joint function remains badly impaired. In osteoarthritis, the knees are usually affected most severely, since they must undergo the constant wear of weight-bearing. If the weight is distributed unevenly on the surfaces of the joints, as is the case with people who are bowlegged or knock-kneed, the damaging effects are accelerated. The best kind of treatment is prevention, but unfortunately, treatment for poorly aligned knees is not so simple. There is a surgical procedure called an osteotomy, performed on the upper end of the tibia or the fibula, which shifts some of the weight to the opposite side of the knee joint, thereby correcting the deformity and enabling the patient to walk without pain. This, of course, is treatment for damage that has already occurred, not preventive. It is hardly conceivable that this operation would appeal to a young person as desirable for preventing of something that might be crippling to him fifty or sixty years in the future. There is one highly important preventive measure available that should be observed by all arthritics, and that is weight control.

One shining exception to the limitations of surgical accomplishment in arthritis is the encouraging percentage of success now being achieved in surgery for arthritis of the hand. This type of surgery has gone beyond the purely reparative status, and is becoming recognized more and more widely as a preventive measure against further damage. Since it has been estimated that there are about five million people in this country with rheumatoid arthritis, of which ninety-four percent have some involvement of their hands, it is not surprising that hand surgery has become a well-recognized specialty. Surgeons who do it usually confine themselves to hand problems alone, finding the human

146

hand a wide enough field to challenge all their expertise.

The intricacies of the bone-joint-tendon structural
mechanism of the hand give it a range of usefulness
without parallel anywhere else in the body. The slight-
est impairment of this harmony of movement can be
devastating to a pianist, in whatever part of the hand
it occurs. Some small disruption of activity, such as the
power to appose the thumb and forefinger, can cause
inefficiency in a great variety of ordinary tasks; complete loss of the use of both hands is probably the most
handicapping destruction the body can suffer. Anything that offers a possibility of averting such a catas-
trophe, therefore, merits widespread attention.

There are two types of attention present-day surgeons give to the arthritic hand. One is the possibility
of removal of the diseased synovial membranes lining
the joints and tendons, which is the site of the destructive process. Results of these synovectomies have been
highly encouraging. Not only has the arthritic pain
been relieved to a remarkable extent, but the destructive process in that area has been halted, thus giving
the synovectomy a preventive role in the treatment of
arthritis.

The age-old clashes of viewpoint between internists and surgeons have their echoes here. The surgeons
say that many of these cases are not referred to them
early enough for optimum results. The internists are
apt to reply (in thought if not in words), "We are being
made the goats for surgical failures." Happily for the
patient, a meeting of the minds is being strived for on
this question. Studies are being made on results
achieved after varying intervals of delay for a trial of
medical treatment. Before referring the patient for sur-

147

gical consideration, some are in favor of setting a period of, say, four or six months, during which medical treatment is allowed a trial. The majority of opinion seems to be, however, that arthritis is too unpredictable for these arbitrary time limits, that each case should be evaluated individually. All this discussion has not been fruitless. It has fixed more firmly in the minds of all concerned persons—internists, surgeons, and patients —that treatment possibilities exist and that it is advisable to use them to the best possible advantage.

The other type of work surgeons do on arthritic hands is the correction of deformities. This calls for a digit-by-digit, or even a joint-by-joint, evaluation, having in mind what corrections will most nearly restore the hand to a useful state. Ghastly deformities will sometimes have occurred, making the hand look like a distorted claw. These are caused by contractures of various tendons, which destroy the nice balance between the flexors and extensors, accompanied at times by rupture of some of the tendons and partial displacement of some of the joints. Combinations of these pathologic developments make possible a variety of deformities, some of which occur with sufficient frequency to constitute patterns that can be given descriptive names. There is the "mallet finger," with the distal phalanx fixed in a right-angled flexion like the head of a hammer. In the "swan neck" deformity, a finger becomes bent in a curve that is graceful in a swan, horrendous in a hand. One of the late developments in the disease is the "ulnar drift," in which the fingers become slanted in a fixed position away from the thumb.

Surgical treatment of the arthritic hand has none of the cut-and-be-done-with-it quality of many other operations, such as an appendectomy or the excision of a tumor. Whatever the pathology in the hand, it is never a complete indication for surgery. The surgeon evaluates not only the hand, but the entire patient, and those for whom surgery is recommended are carefully chosen. Of two patients with similar pathology, surgery may be advised for one and not the other. Many patients are long past any hope of benefit from operative reconstruction. As one authority expresses it: "Not only has the disease destroyed their hand, but it has to a great extent damaged their psyche. They do not have the desire to get well. They do not have proper motivation to follow through postoperatively with the tedious exercises which are absolutely necessary for maximum improvement from operative rehabilitation. In this group of patients operative reconstruction is definitely contraindicated."

Another condition that may deter surgery on the arthritic hand is the atrophy of muscles after long disuse. This may involve muscles of the forearm as well as the hand. Obviously, it would accomplish little to restore the possibility of motion to a long-inert part if the muscles are too weak to supply the power. It has been found advisable to require such patients to demonstrate the regenerative ability of their atrophic muscles before deciding upon surgery. These patients are instructed in a series of exercises to be performed regu-larly for several months. If at the end of that time there is not a definite increase in forearm diameter, and an improvement in the pinch-and-grip power of their deformed hands, the value of surgery for them is considered very questionable.

The selection of patients for reconstructive hand surgery is thus summarized by Drs. Jerome E. Adamson, C. E. Horton, and R. A. Mladick, all of the Norfolk General Hospital of Norfolk, Virginia: "Reconstruction is most effective in those patients who are seen early in the course of the disease, who have not developed disuse atrophy of the forearm and hand musculature, and who still have a postive well-motivated approach toward obtaining improvement."

Much of the surgery for the treatment of the larger arthritic joints involves the use of prostheses, a Greek word meaning "addition," or "substitution." A glass eye, false teeth, a wooden leg, are all protheses of the simpler sort, capable of being added or removed at will. The more complicated prostheses are those incorporated as a permanent part of the body structure. These are in common use by vascular surgeons to replace damaged heart valves or sections of blood vessels. By far the most ambitious prosthesis yet dreamed of, still on the surgical drawing boards, is the mechanical heart, (unless one dares to look shudderingly over the fence of reality at the mechanical brain of science fiction).

Orthopedic surgeons have their own notable accomplishments in this field. For joints rendered useless by the wear-and-tear of disease, for example, "total hip joint replacement" is now a repeatedly successful procedure. Prostheses are being used successfully for knees also. In both these instances, weight-bearing has been a factor in the disintegration of the joints, and this, combined with the disease, results in the literal destruction of the joint properties necessary for function. There is nothing left to be repaired, and replacement is the only solution.

Shortly before this chapter was written I saw a patient who is a notable example of the success of knee prostheses. She had them in both her knees, after having lost the power of locomotion almost completely. Three months after the operation on her right knee, which permitted her to bend and straighten her formerly stiff joint at will, she had surgery on her left knee also, which was almost as badly afflicted as the right had been. When I saw her, about two months later, she was able to rise from her chair without assistance and take a few steps about the room without help of crutches, cane, or walker. She was working assiduously at her own rehabilitation, having set a goal for herself. Her daughter was being married in about six weeks and she was determined to be able to walk down the aisle in the proper manner. I understand that she made it.

Physiotherapy is a large part of the treatment regimen for any kind of arthritis, and again, it is highly individualized. Only one rule applies to everyone, and that is, "Get the advice of your doctor first." What kind of exercise? How much rest? The patient, if left to his own devices, is apt to answer these questions according to his own temperament rather than to his therapeutic advantage. The timid ones, very sensitive to pain, tend to be too inactive, while the more forceful characters may damage themselves in their rebellious determination to "work off" their affliction.

Under only the most extraordinary circumstances does a doctor advise prolonged bed rest for an arthritic. The results could be a secondary affliction as devious to treat as the original arthritis. The fact is that the entire rest-exercise regimen for arthritis is mutually antagonistic. What we seek is the procedure that will do most good with the least damage. It would be wonderfully helpful to allow those inflamed surfaces of sore joints to heal without the irritation of motion or weight-bearing, which would mean keeping them at rest. But alas, this cannot be done because the joints do not move of their own volition. If a joint is to remain at rest, the muscles and ligaments that do the work must also be motionless. Even when the patient is immobilized, they still persist in their defensive duty toward the sore joint by tightening up about it into a protective shield, which, if allowed to remain undisturbed, will eventually become fixed. Thus the joint becomes immovable. Most patients are aware of this stiffening of the muscles about a sore joint when they get up in the morning. After a night's rest it takes them a while to get limbered up.

Exercise may be considered in two categories, active and passive. Active exercise is the simpler of the two, being the kind of exercise the patient can do himself. Even this kind, however, needs some direction. A patient may think smugly, after walking a mile or jogging a few blocks, "Well, I've surely done enough exercise for today," but if the exercise has not involved motion of the muscles about the arthritic area, it does not count as therapy. In other words, exercise for the arthritic must be specialized to his needs if it is to be beneficial. The prescribed activity may be so simple that the patient would scarcely think of it as exercise— such things as a pill-rolling motion of the fingers, clenching and unclenching the fist, slow flexion and extension of an extremity. Daily stretchings of an arm to higher and higher points on a wall is an effective exercise for reducing the stiffness of shoulder muscles from whatever cause, a common one being the sequel to radical breast surgery. Besides relieving stiffness, exercises may also be used to strengthen muscles that have become weakened by inactivity. A type often used for this purpose involves resistance by pushing or pulling against a force, sometimes with the help of weights or springs.

Passive exercises are more complicated, as they require the help of another person. The helper does all the flexing, extending, stretching, lifting of the afflicted part without any active help of the patient, hopefully strengthening the afflicted muscles to the point where the patient can exercise himself.

If an arthritis patient is hospitalized for a time, much can be done for him in the physiotherapy department. Not only can he have his proper exercises under trained supervision, but he will be taught many helpful modalities that he can continue for himself at home. Various types of heat treatment will be available to him. Heat is the oldest known muscle relaxant, and it has never gone out of favor. It eases that protective spasticity about an arthritic joint, relieving pain and soreness. It may be used in various forms, the simplest being the heating pad or hot-water bottle, easy for the patient to manage by himself. Heat may also be supplied by hot packs, lamps, or electric pads. A hot tub bath at home affords solace to many. Other forms of hydrotherapy are available in hospital physiotherapy departments, such as whirlpool baths, which give a soothing massaging action as well as warmth. The entire body may be immersed, and there are also smaller tanks for the treatment of some one afflicted part, such as an arm or a leg.

The extent to which treatment of arthritis may be individualized is endless. Often a patient may be helped by some gambit that has never been published in the extensive literature about the treatment of the disease. The Arthritis Foundation (1212 Avenue of the

Americas, New York, N.Y. 10036—there are subsidiary state chapters) is always on the alert for any new helpful procedure, and every arthritic should have its manual on the home care of arthritis. It explains in detail the programs for rest and exercise and the logic behind them. It cautions patients about the importance of posture and gait, and lists appliances available for self-help in specific instances. However, this manual is by no means a do-it-yourself substitute for professional guidance. It is an adjunct to medical care, helpful to both physician and patient. The physician can find in it a detailed elaboration of much of the advice he gives to his arthritic patients.

A highly important warning to arthritis sufferers in general appears in the introduction of this booklet: "One of the chief dangers is keeping an arthritic joint immobilized. This can lead to deformity and crippling." I have heard a colleague of mine say that the advice he gives most often to his arthritis patients is this two-word sentence, "Keep going."

15

Aids and Adaptations

The natural reaction of a person with an affliction handicapping to his motility is to reach out into his surroundings for physical assistance. He steadies himself against a wall, leans on one piece of furniture after another as he progresses through a room, grasps the friendly arm of a companion. Out of these primal needs have developed a standard series of mechanical aids for the physically handicapped, such as crutches, canes, walkers, wheelchairs, all of which have undergone many revisions to increase their usefulness.

Canes and crutches are always rubber-tipped, to prevent slipping. Canes may be "C"-headed or "T"-headed, fitting the ease of the hand that grasps them. The standard length is thirty-six inches. Crutches need more individual adaptation. They should be made to measure, with padded hand grips and shoulder pieces, made so that most of the weight is borne by the hand grips. Walkers have been improved greatly since they were first devised, now made with lightweight but just as strong material as the early ones so that they can be moved about with greater ease, and fashioned to encircle the body about halfway in order to be equally supportive on both sides. Wheelchairs are constantly being improved, one constant challenge being a decrease in weight without loss in strength. They are cushioned for greater comfort, may be folded easily for transportation by car or plane, and some have been motorized.

Braces and splints have to be adjusted carefully to the individual patient. A splint for arthritis is essentially a lightweight cast, usually made of plaster of Paris, which helps provide rest or protection to an acutely inflamed joint, most often to a wrist, hand, or knee. It may need to be renewed from time to time as the pathological condition changes. The intervals of its use vary, from round-the-clock at first to later broken periods specified by the doctor. Braces may be used to give the extra support needed for motility, or to hold a bony part in optimum alignment.

The feet are often affected in arthritis. In fact it might be said that they are usually affected to some degree in any case of generalized arthritis. This makes well-fitting shoes of great importance. Arthritics should throw style to the winds in the selection of shoes, (and many not-yet-arthritics would profit by following this same advice). Many additions and adaptations are available which make shoes more comfortable to the arthritic foot. A properly fitting Oxford shoe with a straight last and low wide heel is universally advisable. Additional needs may be a metatarsal bar to relieve pressure on the ball of the foot, or a wedge to prevent the foot from turning inward. A springy, padded sole may add much comfort.

Countless aids have been devised for special functions, diminishing the loss of accomplishment for many arthritics, and the list is constantly increasing. The Arthritis Foundation is the best source of information about these. There are long-handled combs and toothbrushes for those whose arthritic shoulders limit their upward reach, long-handled reachers of various kinds, large-handled cups and built-up pencils and eating utensils for arthritic hands with impaired clutching power. All arthritis patients with any impaired function should investigate the possibilities for self-help. Doing things for oneself, decreasing one's dependence upon others, not only improves mobility but builds wonderful morale.

Many modifications may be made in an arthritic's home surroundings to add to his safety and comfort. These are applicable to infirmities from other causes also, including aging. In fact, a large part of the faltering movements of the aged may be due to the stiffness of arthritic joints. Some of these modifications—nonskid pads under loose rugs, railings beside stairs, grabbars above bathtubs—might well be standard equipment for any home, even those occupied by vigorous young people. They would tend to diminish accidents and would make things easier for the elderly visitor.

The shape of a chair can make a great deal of difference to the comfort of an arthritic. One with the seat too low or too deep can be a strain on his back, hips, and knees and be difficult to rise out of. To counteract this, large upholstered chairs may be fortified in the proper places with loose cushions. Straight chairs may have a higher supplemental seat fixed in place, or have the legs fastened to platforms of suitable height. Toilet seats are often too low for the arthritic to use in comfort. For these, removable accessory seats are available.

In my own home I have a one-room-with-bath apartment that is arranged in more detail to the needs of the physically handicapped than any I have seen elsewhere in a private residence.

This apartment was built for our daughter Virginia about fifteen years ago, and as time goes by we have become more and more aware of its importance to all of us. She has been able to continue living at home, which might have become impossible without it.

Her handicap is cerebral palsy, not arthritis, but in the belief that there are a sufficient number of overlaps in the problems of the physically handicapped to make the knowledge helpful to others, I describe it here. The apartment was designed by Virginia herself, with the devoted cooperation of builders, plumbers, electricians, and cabinetmakers. These workmen all said that they were doing some things they had never seen or heard of.

Virginia is more severely handicapped than most arthritics. She has never been able to walk, and she does not synchronize the use of her hands well. She sits in her wheelchair, therefore, only at meals and for transportation, and she cannot operate it herself. Most of her day is spent sitting on the floor, where she reads, operates her television by remote control, uses her electric typewriter, tape recorder, and adding machine. (She keeps all our household accounts.)

She has a built-in bed of the exact height of the seat of her wheelchair, which enables her to slide from chair to bed, or to back off her bed into the chair when it is set into place with the brakes fixed. She can also get into bed from the floor, which has some gentle carpeted terracing on one side to decrease the distance to the bed level. She pulls herself up by a heavy strap attached to the opposite side of the framework of the bed. Getting out of bed is no problem—a low drop to the carpeted surface.

Her bathroom is arranged so that she can use the toilet and bathe herself without help. The lavatory and mirrored cabinet are at floor level. The toilet bowl is set below the floor, so that the seat rests on the floor. The bathtub is sunken, with a long grab-bar on the wall along the far side, and a shorter one along about a third of the near side. She pulls herself out of the tub by another heavy strap welded into the floor. She finds it easier to get out while the tub is still partially full of water, giving some buoyancy to her weight.

This was an expensive project, more so than we had planned upon, and now it would be prohibitive to anyone except those in a much higher income bracket. It is described here because I think I can foresee a time when it might be helpful to a great many people. Apartment housing designed for the physically handicapped is not too far in the future. Such things as I have detailed, when produced in multiples instead of singly, would be much less expensive.

People with physical handicaps have been among the least vociferous and demanding of the minority groups, but even they are now beginning to get some sympathetic attention from the public. For example, there is a growing awareness that a long flight of steps leading to the front door of a public building such as a church or a library may add grandeur in the architect's eye, but it makes the building practically inaccessible to citizens on crutches or in wheelchairs. In 1962 I crossed the Atlantic by ship. Among my fellow passengers was a man in a wheelchair, and I talked to him and his wife about the difficulties they met in travel. They told me they had found it practically impossible to travel by air, as most airlines would not take a passenger thus handicapped. Now these limitations have largely been overcome.

In 1970 my husband and I accompanied our daughter on a trip around the world. It was a tour for the handicapped, directed by the renowned Betty Hoffman of the Evergreen Travel Service in Seattle, who is a pioneer in the promotion of travel possibilities for the handicapped and whose expertise on that subject is without equal. Traveling with her and hearing her discuss the travel problems she had to meet taught me most of what I know about the exigencies to be met by those with some impairment of normal motor functions. Long flights of steps, of course, are a deterrent anywhere, but less so on a trip like this than in one's home town. On an organized tour such as Betty Hoffman's was, an adequate number of porters is always at hand for lifting and carrying when necessary. There are steps, however, that baffle the experts, such as those at the Taj Mahal. They are too steep and narrow for the safety of any but the sure-footed, ambulating under their own power. One of the most unexpectedly arduous bits of travel we met in the entire six weeks was the crossing of a large cobblestone-paved courtyard in Istanbul. There was no way to bypass it, no smooth route over it, by sidewalk or path. It was a trying experience for everyone, whether on crutches, riding in wheelchairs, or pushing them.

One must be knowledgeable about the selection of hotels for the handicapped, Betty told us. She had made several similar trips before ours and had learned most of the deficiencies that can be found in hostelries. A most common one is a bathroom door too narrow to admit a wheelchair. A steep, high threshold between the room and bathroom is another structural idiosyncrasy that can rule out a lodging place. Some hotels have met this problem with hastily constructed removable ramps to be placed one on each side of the threshold. They are usable in an emergency, but not ideal.

Human apathy is another obstruction to be met by any innovation, and the idea of handicapped people traveling about the country a long way from home is a new one to most people. Cooperation in such unheard-of activity requires some mental adjustment and often some outside stimulation, which Betty is adept at supplying. I wondered sometimes if anyone has ever heard her admit, "It can't be done." In Hong Kong, our hotel had a dining room on the top floor with a marvelous view of the island and harbor. The elevator, however, came only to the floor below, with a flight of steps to complete the ascent. One evening several of us went up to the dining room ahead of the main group, telling the maître d'hôtel who met us at the top of the stairs that we did not wish to be seated yet, as we were a part of the handicapped group and would wait for the others. He shook his head vociferously, saying that we had made a mistake, that it was the dining room on the floor below us that we wanted, and pointing to the stairs as proof of the dining room's inaccessibility to any but the able-bodied. Before he had finished talking, the first contingent of our group was coming up the stairs, carried briskly by the porters, and while he watched, agape, all the rest arrived and were assembled ready to dine within a period of ten minutes.

In Japan we found the most all-out effort that I have seen for the comfort of travelers disadvantaged by physical handicaps. This was a building in Osaka, where the World's Fair had just opened, built by the Lions Clubs of Japan, labeled "Services for the Handicapped." Approaches to the building were by easy ramps, and there was an elevator for connection with the monorail on the level above. There was an English-speaking staff in attendance—several men at the business desk and a flock of girls in uniform, all of whom devoted themselves assiduously to the needs of visiting travelers. The girls served tea to everyone, helped any of the women who needed help in the bathroom, arranged tables and chairs for the serving of the box lunches our hotel in Kyoto had packed for us. There were rows of about a hundred wheelchairs ready for lending. In addition to the permanent staff, members of the Osaka Lions Clubs had assigned themselves tours of duty at the building, so that several of them were available to assist travelers in getting to the places they wanted to visit, and to help push the wheelchairs en route.

16

The Role of Psychiatry
in Arthritis

One of the many developments that have taken place in my lifetime is the coming of age of psychiatry. It was a puny infant in my medical school days, with little indication of the directions in which it would mature. Our textbook (I have forgotten the name of the author) was by far the slimmest volume on the shelf of the students' books. True, such names as Freud, Adler, and Jung were in the public eye, but were too controversial and perhaps too poorly understood to be put into a textbook for students. What we were taught was an ironclad classification of the psychoses. I was imbued with the idea that every patient with sufficient mental derangement to be called crazy had to fit into one of these categories—or else. Fitting them in did call for some minor adjustments at times; a magnification of some findings, a toning down of others. By the time we passed the course, we were supposed to be able to make a diagnosis from a given case history. Which is it—schizophrenia, senile dementia, or manic depressive psychosis? It had to be one of them; there was nothing in between for us to consider.

Mistakes in diagnosis were made occasionally, we learned, even by the experts. The most incontrovertible evidence was if a patient got well. If a patient recovered from such a malady as schizophrenia, it was evident that the diagnosis had been wrong in the first place. What, then, was the purpose of studying psychiatry? Pure academics. We had to be as learned in mental disease as in all the physical kinds, didn't we? It may be that the intent of the instruction in psychiatry was not as I have reported it. But it is what I, an average student, got out of it.

Our instruction was not limited to book work by any means. We spent several afternoons of that semester in the wards of a mental institution located in our city. On these wards we saw many of the things we had been reading about—the ravings of mania, the soddenness of depression, the abject posturing of catatonia. We absorbed also the basics of mental disease treatment of that day—lock up the patients and keep them from injuring themselves or others.

It does not behoove any generation of physicians to adopt a harshly critical attitude toward the errors of our predecessors. We should learn from their mistakes but be tolerant in our judgment, as we hope future generations will be tolerant of us. Still, I sometimes find it almost impossible to condone the old classification of "hysteria" as a disease entity. Far too much was shoveled into it. I am convinced that this catchall category often contained cases of the most intense suffering.

In the more humane light of present knowledge,

one shudders to read of all the ills that were disposed of under this heading, and "disposed of" is the best way to put it. The word itself was an unfortunate choice for the name of a disease. It has the connotation of "putting on an act," of a conscious intent to bamboozle somebody to gain sympathy. True, such things happen. Then let the diagnosis apply to them alone. It was the inclusion of so many other things that I deplore.

Among these "hysterical" phenomena were persistent tremors, paralyses, severe contractures of various muscle groups, spasms, convulsions, disturbances of sensation, joint swellings and fixations. Some of these signs might last for months or even years. These cases were baffling to physicians, of course, most of whom directed their endeavors toward "curing" these surface manifestations of trouble, leaving the hidden source undisturbed, except for those few equipped to try some psychoanalysis.

Baffling as these cases were, they were not particularly worrisome to the physician. Uppermost in his mind he carried the assurance "There is no organic pathology here." Therefore these illnesses could not kill anybody. Couldn't they? And didn't they?

It seems to me logical to assume that these so-called weaklings, the "hysterical" ones, were often the strong ones instead, that their physical signs were the expression of their determination to resist whatever was threatening them, of the fight they were putting up. When psychological suffering becomes completely intolerable, the way out often involves a choice between two alternatives, psychosis and suicide.

Psychiatry had tough going in its early years. It had little support, sometimes actual opposition, from other branches of the profession, who tended to relegate it to the same category as astrology, parapsychology, and science fiction. This was especially true of surgeons (I have two in my immediate family) whose credo, "I gotta see it to believe it," is backed up by the pathologists.

The distance from that concept to the present one is another measure of the advance of psychiatry. Now there are few diseases (I do not think of any, at the moment) that do not have a need for psychological adjustments, sometimes, as a part of their therapeutic regimen, even arthritis, or especially arthritis. Every text on arthritis has a discussion of the psychological factors that are at least, *possible* contributory causes if not direct ones. The most recent symposium on arthritis that I attended had one of the leading psychiatrists of our state, Dr. Sidney L. Sands, on its teaching staff. Now even surgeons are beginning to mellow. Recently I heard a surgeon say that he thought some of the symptoms he had been having were psychosomatic. Psychiatry has come into its own.

Some years ago a member of a local church board told me why one applicant for their pastorate had been crossed off their list, summarily. He had asked whether there was a psychiatrist in the area, and said he could not accept a pastorate in a place where he could not get the psychiatric counseling he needed. The board had been dismayed to realize that he was talking about counseling for *himself,* not his parishioners, which would have seemed sufficiently flagrant to them. Our church boards would probably react in the same way today. A man of God is not supposed to be tortured by human uncertainties. But if anyone doubts that any human being can find himself in the boat of the mentally troubled, I cite the suicide rate in various branches of the medical profession—it is highest among psychiatrists.

Psychiatry has stepped off its aloof academic pedestal and seeks to be a benefactor of mankind. The demand for its services has been phenomenal, far greater than anyone expected. The experience of a small clinic in my state is an example. "We wondered at first whether we had enough work for a psychiatrist," one of the staff said. "Now we have two, and could use another one."

In my rural midwestern state, the sprinkling of psychiatrists is pretty thin. Most of our individual counseling, in mental clinics and in institutions, is done by psychologists. I have come to know quite a number of them secondhand, through their contacts with my patients, and have developed a high regard for them. In itself, psychology seems to attract a special kind of person who genuinely feels involved in other people's troubles. Nothing takes the place of the meeting of minds that must be the basis of successful counseling. "He's my best friend!" an underprivileged little boy told me with glowing face about an older boy who had talked with him about some problems—a one sentence recommendation for any psychologist to treasure. One of the greatest advances is that a large percentage of the work now being done in psychic medicine involves patients who, in the early days, would not have been considered ill. The line of demarcation between the mentally sick and the mentally well is rapidly disappearing. The newer concept is that we are all in the same boat, and our differences are only a matter of degree and of our ability to cope. Attention is increasingly directed to the earlier and comparatively minor mental problems, things that may be only nagging in their present state but which have a growth potential that could lead to disaster. There is no way of foretelling which symptoms have such potential; any persistently troubling ones should be considered hazardous. Worries that ravage one's sleep night after night; the headache the follows a family argument on a certain subject; the upset stomach when relatives are due for an unavoidable visit; fears that insist upon holding a conference in the early morning hours; unforgettable remorse over something in the past; stiffening about a joint in protest against a confrontation that cannot be avoided; burning in the throat and stomach concomitant with job insecurity—the list is endless. According to these criteria, who is sick and who is well? Who has not suffered some of these "mental symptoms"? Years ago when I was new in practice, I used to tell women patients who were worried about the signs of aging, "The best way I know to keep from looking your age is to be born feebleminded." Weak minds make few records.

Realization of this universality of mental problems has taken away most of the stigma that used to be attached to psychiatric treatment. Going to a psychiatrist has been common and even fashionable for some time in urban centers, but in my rural area some of that old feeling remains. A referral to a psychiatrist is a duty for which the general practitioner must often summon all his tact and diplomacy. There are times when most of us come up lacking. With my best efforts, I have had patients react the full scale, from dismayed to infuriated. As might be surmised, the worst reactors are apt to be those in greatest need.

Physicians still have to be constantly on their guard against making too hasty a diagnosis of psychosomatic origins, always a last ditch stand. Once backed into that position, the doctor stops looking for organic pathology; therefore he must not back into it too soon, not until after every possible organic cause has been explored and ruled out. No matter how certain he may feel that he won't find anything, he has to keep looking, piling up myriads of tests and examinations with negative findings. I should not attempt to estimate how many X rays I have ordered for what I felt certain were "nervous stomachs." But feeling is not proof, and one must have proof, not only for one's own peace of mind but to convince the patient. The patient always believes his trouble is organic, and it is sometimes difficult to convince him otherwise. "Only a cancer could make me feel this bad," is the judgment of many a troubled mind. All of which makes psychosomatic illnesses difficult and time-consuming just from the diagnostic angle alone, even before getting into the treatment. There is probably no one of us who has not erred, who has not called symptoms psychic that were later found to have a well-defined organic basis, plain and clear, once the probings were turned to the right direction. These are among the cases a doctor never forgets.

Many years ago I heard a lecture by a famous surgeon, whose name would be familiar to anyone reading this book. Before X-ray techniques had been developed to their present accuracy, one of his patients was a man who complained of persistent distress in his epigastrium (the upper-middle part of the abdomen, just below the breastbone). He was a jumpy, edgy sort of person, who might easily be suspected of having psychosomatic symptoms. This doctor, besides being an astute and skillful surgeon himself, was a member of the staff of a famous clinic, where, according to well-based popular opinion, nothing is ever neglected or over-looked. All their tests and examinations, however, failed to uncover any organic pathology.

"You mean it's all in my head?" the man asked.

"In a manner of speaking, yes," the surgeon replied, and the patient left, looking neither happy nor convinced.

In about two months he came back again, bringing a handful of gallstones to show the surgeon. "These didn't come out of my head," he told the doctor. He had consulted another surgeon, who did not demand proof, but was willing to operate on suspicion.

Emanuel Miller reports one case history that refutes the too-ready assumption of psychological sources in low-back pain. A man of forty complained of intense pain in the area of his sacrum and coccyx (the lower extremity of the spinal column). His coccyx was removed, without relief. He continued to have as much pain in the sacrum, just above the coccyx. No organic basis for it was found, and since he appeared to be a somewhat hysterical type, anyway, he was referred for psychiatric treatment which included hypnosis. Meanwhile he developed a persistent cough, and X ray showed a lung malignancy. He died, an autopsy was done, and malignant metastases were found in his sacrum. (One wonders about the discomfiture of the psychiatrist if this was one of the cases which he considered due to guilt feelings about masturbation!)

One big reason why arthritics do not get all the psychological attention they ought to have is that they are not asking for it. Quite the reverse. They tend to have a defensive, hands-off attitude, making it difficult to pry psychological data out of them. Their response is apt to be something like, "It's my arthritis that bothers me, doctor. What do my business worries, my sex life, or my other family problems have to do with it?" No wonder that a busy doctor is tempted to take them at their word and lay off the subject.

Does Everybody Need an Analyst? is the title of a book by psychiatrist William G. Stone. Not everybody does, he admits, and he proposes a scale by which each individual can measure his own level of security, a sort of do-it-yourself appraisal of his own emotional status.

I believe strongly that a person should take some responsibility upon himself for his own mental health needs. His first reaction to troubling tensions should not be to run panicking to a psychiatrist. He should lie on his *own* couch at home and do some thinking first. It will be a lot cheaper, and he won't have to wait for an appointment. Then if he cannot reason things out for himself, if he finds that his thinking is only burrowing him more deeply into his quagmire of fears and worries, then, by all means, he should seek professional help. But even so, his preliminary thinking may afford some clarifying data to the psychiatrist.

Does every arthritic need a psychological appraisal? The answer is yes, and most patients who have consulted a physician at all have already had such an appraisal, probably without being aware of it. Some psychological estimate is registered automatically in a physician's mind with every patient he sees. It is almost subconscious with him, something he couldn't help if he tried. In any interview he cannot avoid arriving at some conclusions about the patient's intelligence, truthfulness, reliability, mental stability, and the genuineness of his symptoms. Probably none of this goes into his records unless there is something glaringly out of line with the norm he has fixed in his mind.

The scope of possible psychiatric involvement in the care and supervision of arthritics is a wide one. It may (but seldom does) include therapy sessions in a psychiatrist's office. As do most other modes of treatment, psychotherapy has its best chance of success in the early stages of the disease before the occurrence of organic structural damage. It may also be useful later, in the minimizing of acute flare-ups. Knowledgeable authorities are apt to insert a warning in their discussions of psychiatric treatment, to the effect that any deeper-conflict problems should be approached only by the highly skilled. A know-it-all amateur or a reckless innovator may possess a terrifying power of destruction, unrealized until the occurrence of some calamity, such as suicide.

According to the findings of Dr. Samuel B. Guze of Washington University, researchers have found that from five to fifty percent of their cases of systemic lupus erythematosus, SLE for short, have had the most serious psychiatric complications. Some of these have involved both repeated hospitalizations for the psychological problems alone, and expert care by psychiatrists. However, SLE is by no means a typical picture of the role of psychiatry in arthritis. The great majority of people with arthritis never need the attention of either a psychiatrist or a psychologist which is fortunate, as there wouldn't be enough of such expertise to go around. Yet they do need some psychological support, and I like to believe that most of them have it available to them, if they are not too stubborn and standoffish to accept it. The concept of psychotherapy should be broad enough to include anything that alters the mental condition for the patient; which makes possible psychotherapists out of everybody in close contact with him.

I have known people among personnel in the physiotherapy department of a hospital, both men and women, who contributed as much to the mental as to the physical well-being of their patients. I recall one woman badly crippled with arthritis on her morning trip to physiotherapy. In her room, she got about on crutches, but for this long trip down the hall from the elevator she was in a wheelchair. This was not a good morning for her. She had news from the farm that one of the cows was sick, and a hard rain had flooded some of the corn. The nurse said she was crying at breakfast time and did not eat much. The therapist on duty this morning was a young woman. She greeted the patient by name, with a smile. She remembered from which side it was easier to help the patient from her wheelchair, exclaimed with pleasure to note that the left knee seemed a little less stiff than it had been yesterday. Throughout the passive exercises she was considerate of the pain threshold, yet gently insistent, and praised the patient for her fortitude. "Together we are going to get somewhere" was the feeling in the air throughout the session, and at the end of it the patient left with a smile and with a new vigor in her bearing.

The family physician is, of course, the most obvious and most nearly constant arbiter of the arthritic patient's welfare. His helpfulness is as varied as his own personality traits, as well as those of his patients, and the permutations of his inspiration. What the patient is asking may be very simple and direct: "something to take" for his joints, but the physician's responsibility goes much farther than that. In addition to the direction of the obvious medical therapy, it is usually up to him to decide when the patient would profit by consulting an orthopedist, surgeon, psychiatrist, or whatever specialist seems indicated.

The family physician's own therapy must include much of a psychological nature, his close association with the patient insures this. No amount of scientific learning can take the place of a sympathetic attitude. Sympathy is not just an isolated emotion, but a force which cannot fail to direct him to seek out ways of helping the patient. The doctor teams up with the patient in the determination that neither of them must accept defeat. The patient, knowing that he is hitched to a forceful teammate, that he is not "going it alone," can hardly fail to be stimulated to greater endeavors on his own behalf.

A very valuable therapeutic tactic is offering all the possible encouragements—improvements that are within the realm of probability; accomplishments of other people with similar handicaps; possibilities open to each patient for a useful life. Any of these may put the light of hope into an otherwise darkened life. These are cited as a part of the family doctor's regimen because he is most apt to be aware of them, but they could be supplied by anyone else with similar knowledge.

Mental health groups throughout the country are doing a great deal toward reaching incipient mental problems before they diversify, erode, and possibly inflict damages that later will need prolonged psychiatric study and treatment. The shortcut in any kind of therapeutics is to keep little problems from becoming big ones. One activity of the mental health groups is to hold all-day meetings for group discussion of the problems of modern living. These are open to the public—any interested person may come—and the entire assemblage is then subdivided into smaller groups, each with a moderator of some medical or psychological background.

At one such meeting I attended, the catchy discussion title for one of these subgroups was "Growing Old with Style," and the staff could not understand why I objected to it. I had difficulty in explaining it myself. "Style" has always been a touchy word with me. It is a lovely word when used in the sense of an individual characteristic, a distinctive trait—the style of an artist, a writer, or a musician is something that belongs to him or her alone. But it has another meaning almost exactly the opposite to this, which I find abhorrent—"style" used in the sense of "in the popular fashion." Here it is too closely related to "conformity," which is about as spineless a recommendation as I can think of.

Conform! Conform! The most stultifying demand made on the human race. Yet few of us do anything but accede to it. Worse still, we pass along the pressure to younger generations to do the same; and the nearer and dearer the individuals involved, the more importunate become our pressures. We never question our own qualifications to give advice to the young. "Why can't you be more like your brother Sid, or your Uncle Malcolm?" The cry of protest, "But I'm not like that!" if unheeded, may become the advance bugle of rebellion, peaceful or otherwise.

Or, if the human machine lacks the will of rebellion or exercises all its power of restraint against it, resentment may be retained indefinitely to cause any number of possible impairments of function. The moral: an unhampered control system is the best guarantee for a long and happy life of the human machine.

If there is a home situation that contributes to the unrest of an arthritic, sometimes a social worker can detect this most easily. Her training has made her acutely sensitive to family dysrhythmias. Ministers are in a position to give valuable family counseling, and they are probably the ones most patients turn to first. There is no way of estimating their contribution to the mental health of their congregation but I am certain it is a large one.

There have been reports in the literature of highly successful treatment of arthritis by psychiatry alone. It seems that these cases must have been exceptional, that the best use of psychiatry in arthritis is as an adjunctive treatment, combined with medicine or surgery, or both. Good teamwork among the right doctors is the best answer. Psychiatry alone would certainly be stymied in the type of case in which organic damage has already occurred—fixed muscle contractures, joint erosions, and so on. Even in such cases, psychotherapy could conceivably turn off the malign stimuli and make a protective barrier about the damaged tissue, thus preventing further damage. But to expect the disease to be psyched into backing up and going away, taking its accumulated debris with it, is too tall an order.

A question that naturally arises in a reader's mind is "Whom should I consult if I have symptoms that suggest I may have this disease?" I have heard such a question asked only recently. "What kind of doctor should I go to? A psychiatrist, an orthopedic surgeon, an internist, or a family doctor?"

My suggestion would be to cross the first two off the list immediately, as primary consultants. This is not downgrading them in the least; it is what they themselves would prefer. As is reiterated over and over in any discussion of arthritis, this is a systemic disease, not limited to joints. These specialists would prefer that some general work be done first, to make sure there is something about the case pertinent to their field. The psychiatrist also wants to know what organic pathology is present and what part it plays in the symptoms. As stated in another chapter, most orthopedic surgery, except in accident cases, is done only after an intensive preliminary study which involves the entire picture of the disease. So, as a general rule, it is better for an arthritic to be seen first by someone who is accustomed to looking at patients as individual wholes, one who does not limit himself to a specialty. Later, the doctor may need to send the patient out beyond his own horizons, but at least he will know in which direction to send him. There are exceptions to this rule, as to all others. It is conceivable for an arthritic to present such alarming coincidental psychotic symptoms that he needs to be seen by a psychiatrist immediately. But for a patient with a tendon contracture severe enough to prevent his walking, surgery would be a paramount need.

17

What You Can Do

The final chapter in this book on arthritis should be dedicated to the woman in her late eighties who, after reading my book about heart disease, told her daughter, "But she didn't tell me what to *do!*" In other words, I had not given this heart patient the idea that I had anything to say to her, personally. Whatever the book meant to anyone else, in her case I had to admit it was a miserable failure.

In this book I am trying to do better. The information in it, the historical data, and the scientific dissertations are merely the necessary authenticating background for what most of the book's readers really want to know. Practically all the readership attracted to this book will be people who have arthritis themselves or have someone in their family who does.

What these readers are looking for, therefore, must surely be the ways in which the scientific information contained herein touches them personally, its pointed application to their own needs. "What does this mean to me?" "How does this apply to my case?" "How will it help me?" "What should I be doing about *my* arthritis?"

So you have arthritis? Or someone in your family has it? As you already know, you are one of many thousands. Perhaps that knowledge has comforted you somewhat at times. A patient with cerebral palsy once told me that reading about others with her disease always boosted her morale with the message "You are not alone."

The arthritis you have in common is only one fine connecting thread among a great mass of people who branch off from it in an endless variety of characteristics. Even your arthritis differs widely. If you are one whose trouble started as an acute attack of rheumatoid arthritis, or gout, or spondylitis, or any of the other sharply defined diseases of the group, in the classical manner, than you have doubtless already seen a doctor and had some advice. All well and good. Follow it. Your questions are probably being answered as they arise.

You may be one of the many whose symptoms have not been so clear-cut. Their very vagueness causes questions to arise in your mind. Is anything the matter with you at all, you wonder. You certainly wouldn't say you are sick. Still, you know you feel quite a lot different from the way you used to. The change has been so gradual that you have to look back quite a way to detect it. Physical work seems to make you more tired. You don't feel as supple and graceful as you used to. Exercising was no more to you than a colt frolicking in a meadow. Now you notice it—not right away, perhaps, but that night or the next day. You even notice the activity of getting out of bed. Preposterous, it seems to you, when you think about it. You are not old enough to be feeling like this, you tell yourself indignantly.

If you can identify any of this malaise as an actual stiffness, especially about any certain joints, or if you have had an aching in any joints, you will certainly have thought of arthritis. One exception to this generality occurs to me, however. If this pain or aching is in the joints where the lower jaw hooks onto the skull, you probably thought it was some kind of ear trouble. Nobody ever expects to get arthritis there, but it can happen.

What should you do? Your own inclination will veer you toward one or the other of two extremes, according to the personality make-up we have been talking about. You can decide to ignore the whole business, or you can go overboard in the other direction. Hopefully you will find a spot for yourself between these two extremes, preferably a little nearer the first one. Not that you should ignore your symptoms by any means. But do take a calm view of them. Make an assessment of what you can recall about the earliest manifestations of your trouble. To help you do this, get the booklets your Arthritis Foundation (there is a chapter somewhere in your vicinity) will be glad to send you, free.

Now to the look at yourself. Had you had any other illness recently? Had you been working extra hard, and if so, what parts of your body had been put under the extra strain? Arms and shoulders, from pulling down heavy books or other objects from high shelves? Does your job involve back strain? One mechanic developed severe arthritis of the spine, after years of spending most of his working day on his back under cars. Is it your neck that is stiff and painful? Like that of a secretary who sat at a desk all day and twisted her neck at frequent intervals to use the adding machine behind her. Perhaps your lower extremities have been taking extra punishment. Have you been kneeling a lot, say from working in your garden? Or eating too much, making your knees suffer from your weight? The ankles are vulnerable to strains, also. A patient of mine took up jogging when it became popular, with the over enthusiasm a beginner is apt to display. She was a little too heavy for her rather fragile bony structure, and after two weeks she came in with badly swollen and painful ankles. You could go on from here, and if you come up with anything that seems pertinent, it will suggest its own moves toward remedial action.

Now this may come harder to you. Look into your own mind. Don't flinch! Improvement of your general mental health is a part of your protection against arthritis, and it could even affect your arthritis directly. Who knows? Like a cold shower, you'll feel better after than during. So into it!

Are you worrying about something you never talk to anybody about? That's the worst kind. Are you ashamed of something, blaming yourself for something —such as a mean, jealous feeling that you can't get out of your system? Have you had a grief or a disappointment that you are afraid you will never get over? Are you so discouraged over your outlook in life that you are actually depressed? Does "it," whatever it is, keep you awake at night? If so, sleeping pills are no solution, as you have probably found. "It" is always waiting for you when you wake up. In general, being slugged to sleep at night with one kind of pill and kicked into action in the morning with another is a heck of a way to live.

Besides, lying awake sometimes at night is not so terrible as many people think. After all, it is a good time to think. People can sometimes get their best creative ideas in the middle of the night. So try to train yourself to think creatively, not destructively. Point your thoughts toward a solution of your problems, rather than let them run around in circles like rats in a cage. It will be difficult, but try it anyway. It will be a good mental exercise that may eventually bring results.

If you are one of those at the other end of the personality spectrum, who easily becomes completely engrossed in "taking care of yourself," then all these previous admonitions apply to you too—with a few additions. Keeping yourself fit is a worthy ambition, but your *purpose* in doing so should take priority. To keep yourself comfortable, able to go on breathing and eating for a long, long life? Until you can think of better reasons than these, you have not justified your existence. "What good am I?" should be one of your mental prods. Are you a benefit to your environment in any way? Do you accomplish anything? Is anyone better off for having you around? Unless there is some question of this sort to which you can answer yes, then you had better get busy. Your contribution need not be a physical one. Many physically handicapped people have glowing minds that radiate light all about them. Even if you have a simple, unselfish concern for other people, so that they feel they can turn to you for comradeship and understanding, you can be one of the great nourishing factors of society.

Having pinpointed some justification for your deep concern about your health, let's get back to these early symptoms of arthritis. You should arm yourself with some authentic information.

Being one of those who can get wrapped up in

183

concern for your own health, you are probably a precisionist in general. We doctors all have a few patients who jolt us occasionally by the exactitude with which they follow directions, who regard our advice as a holy dictate to be followed blindly, at all costs. People who interpret "q.4.h." as "every four hours" to the point of setting the alarm to waken them on the dot, or who, having a laxative medication prescribed for them, will continue it faithfully almost to the point of flushing themselves down the drain.

If you are such a person, a few words in general before getting back to specifics. There is no piece of advice so fine-tuned that it does not need occasional adjustments for individuals. You should look at every medical direction, therefore, in the light of those invisible "ifs," "provideds" and "unlesses" that accompany it. If the platitude "There are exceptions to every rule" bores you, here is something more colorful: "Salt with commonsense before swallowing."

For arthritis, one doctor's previous mentioned piece of advice was "Keep going." There are plenty of exceptions to this. "Keep going" is a forceful way of saying, "Don't let the muscles and tendons about those sore joints remain inactive long enough to stiffen permanently into contractures, or you will be a lot worse off than you are now." It does *not* mean, "Keep going, even if the pain of motion nearly kills you."

The subject of pain warrants some discussion at this point. People can be sissies about pain, but a healthy respect for pain is not a weakness. It can be the better part of valor. Pain is the oldest alarm system in existence; it evolved with us, from the time we developed a brain to house the reception center. Pain in any part of the body should never be ignored. It should be inves-

184

tigated and explained as quickly as possible. Only after this is done is the physician willing to short-circuit it with pain-relieving medication.

The pain of arthritis is often self-explanatory. Moving a certain joint hurts. To keep on doing it, then, seems asinine. Here is where judgment and common sense come into play. While keeping it motionless feels best, inactivity over an *extended* period is *verboten*, so we seek the best medium solution—exercise of the surrounding muscles and tendons to keep them pliable, while causing the least possible pain to the sore joint. Some doctors now even advocate keeping arthritis patients in selected cases bedfast for restricted intervals, a procedure that was formerly frowned upon.

If you have had your arthritis a long time, or are a rather impatient person in general, you have probably had periods of dissatisfaction with what your doctor has been doing for you. In every paper or magazine you pick up you see ads for things to be done for arthritis that sound a lot more promising than what is being done for you. Promising is the key word, often the distinguishing one between quackery and authenticity. But in your frame of mind, you are discouraged and bored, ready to meet some dazzling bamboozlement more than half way. You promise yourself you will be cautious and sensible. You wouldn't think of letting yourself be sold on something that does sound rather outlandish, without the recommendation of someone who has tried it, or the advice of friends. But neither of these will be hard to find. If the first person you ask doesn't come across with what you want to hear, you keep looking until you find one that does.

Although you would not admit it even to yourself, you are not looking for advice, really. You are looking

185

for someone who will back you up in something you have already decided to do—at which point you are ripe for the plucking.

Assuming the sad likelihood that you are one of those whom no amount of advice is going to save completely, then let us consider the worst contingency first. Whatever else you do, *don't* take medications that your own doctor has not prescribed. *Do* believe that no one has any efficient and safe medicine that he doesn't know about. A "new" medicine may seem fine at first, make you feel so much better that you are willing to throw all caution to the winds. But you have no concept of the damages it may do to you upon prolonged use. If you are determined to be a sucker, do jump into one of these other booby traps I shall mention, by preference, much as I hate to see you do it. Worthless is less bad than dangerous.

If you are fixed in your determination to "try something else," there is a strong likelihood that you have something specific in mind. You know somebody, maybe a close friend whose honesty and sagacity you would swear to, whose arthritis has been definitely better since she started to use this new whatever-it-is. Let's say it is an electrical gadget to be strapped about a sore joint. Before you go and buy likewise, why don't you survey the market for arthritis "cures"? Your association with this particular friend has pinpointed your attention unduly in one direction. By shopping around you will learn that there are many other scientific marvels, attested to by many other honest, well-meaning people, that guarantee (almost) to cure your arthritis. The longer you look, the more you will find, and knowing these things will make you think, maybe even teach you something.

186

Group therapy has become one of our modern ways of life. It sometimes affords a salubrious give-and-take, very bolstering to the morale. You can have a form of group therapy for your arthritis also. One of its appeals is that a nice trip is a part of it. If you are lonely and tired, discouraged and aching, the dazzle of the trip might very well blind you to the dankness of your destination, an abandoned mine eighty-five feet underground, where you sign up for a series of fifteen sittings at several dollars each. Yes, there is actually such a place as this, doing a good business, the last I heard. There is one possible way that I can think of for you to be benefited from these seances: they will provide a diversion from the humdrum aspects of your arthritis.

I hope all these negative things I am saying will not make you think I am putting you down, that those who qualify for this advice are the lunatic fringe of arthritics, less balanced and intelligent than most. The exact opposite is true. You are the great majority: it has been estimated that ninety percent of all arthritics at some time fall prey to one quack cure or another.

So nothing is left to you, then, except resignation to your fate? "I'm fed up with this dog-in-the-manger attitude! If doctors can't cure my arthritis, they ought to be willing for me to try something else!"

At this point we both admit that you are feeling pretty downcast, at a dead end of your hopes. Now is the time for you to nudge yourself, to stop looking down. Look backward, for a start, at how many other diseases, much more lethal than any form of arthritis, have finally succumbed to the same patient, persistent probing methods of attack that are now being used against arthritis.

On my first day of school in Audubon, Iowa, I was

sent home because I had not yet been vaccinated against smallpox. Now this disease has been so nearly exterminated in this country that the stringent requirements for universal vaccination are being lifted.

In a town where I once lived was an elderly couple who were considered very odd. They were childless, did not associate much with other people, appeared to have few interests or diversions. Then one day I learned something about their early history and understood them much better! They had had five children, who had all died of diphtheria in one six-week period. How frantic and despairing these parents must have felt at the impotence of the treatment the medical profession then had to offer. Now, when did you last hear of anyone dying of diphtheria or even getting it? And what has caused it to disappear from the scene? Not some easy-way opportunist with visions of dollar signs dancing in his head, but the same plodding, persistent medical profession that is now plodding just as persistently after arthritis.

Everyone knows that research is the road to discovery of the causes and cures and that research costs money. But we need to revise some of our thinking about the money being spent for research on arthritis. In the late 1960's it was estimated that about fifteen million dollars a year was being spent on arthritis research. But how big does it sound beside the three to four hundred million dollars that is being spent every year for arthritis quackery? This is money wasted, poured down the drain, with results that vary from useless to dangerous.

Another enlightening comparison may be made between this sum being spent for ultimate prevention and cure, and the staggering amount the depredations of the disease are costing this country every year at the present time. Quoting the Arthritis Foundation 1971 annual report: "The total cost to the national economy is estimated to be nearly four billion dollars annually . . . More than twelve million work days are lost each year because of arthritis. This makes the disease second only to respiratory ailments as the leading cause of industrial absenteeism."

If all costs could be measured in dollars, and the allocation of funds for medical research were under the control of financial experts, it seems probable that arthritis eradication would have priority over that of all other diseases. No other disease costs the country so much. What level-headed businessman would consider a piddling fifteen million dollars an adequate sum to invest in a dam against this yearly drain of three and a half billion dollars of medical and disability costs, plus another three to four hundred million spent on the pitiful delusions of quack cures?

Money can be measured but suffering cannot. Arthritis is probably the most torturing disease in existence, considering the aggregate number of people afflicted, their length of life, and the number of days of pain for each. Estimates such as this, however, are vague. They lack the authority of figures that can be expressed in totals. Death is the incontrovertible statistic, and arthritis is not a killer. This automatically has given priority to such diseases as diphtheria, smallpox, poliomyelitis, and cancer in our efforts toward eradication. Under the threat of death, we pay whatever ransom is required. Although financial costs of disease are thus relegated to second place in importance, they should by no means be ignored.

Look about you in your own contemporary world,

189

and do some serious thinking about it and how it has treated you. Are you really the most afflicted person on earth, as you get to thinking sometimes? You have arthritis. If you could make a deal in diseases, what would you trade it for? Multiple sclerosis? No, this kind of crippling may involve mind as well as body. Emphysema? And be hampered by your breathing instead of your joints? A bad bargain. A defective heart, or diabetes, with their constant threats hanging over you? I haven't even mentioned cancer.

Perhaps you could even consider the good aspects of arthritis, as rated among diseases in general. In the first place, it won't kill you. Don't say, "I wish it would" —you know you don't mean it. (The few who *have* meant it and taken steps in that direction are a very very small minority.) Another favorable quality of arthritis is that however much it may torture your body, it leaves your mind alone. True, I have set down herein a number of mental effects of arthritis, but these are all secondary ones. They are not due to the direct deteriorating effect of arthritis on brain tissue, but to your reactions to your disease, some or all of which you could help, if you tried hard enough. In other words, if you have become morose, depressed, irascible, hostile, irritable, and hard to live with *since* you have had arthritis, you have done it to yourself. If you have lost control of your emotions, don't blame the disease. A final quality that makes arthritis a little less difficult to live with is those blessed remissions that most arthritics have, those times when life may seem even a little more worth living.

Now I refer again to that two-word piece of advice, "Keep going." I have cited exceptional cases in which it should not be taken too literally in a physical sense.

190

But no matter in what bad shape your joints are, you can keep going in your mind. Don't let yourself slump into a worthless lump of organic matter. You can think as well as ever. Look for ways to contribute something to your environment. Make yourself as light a burden as possible to your family. Keep yourself alert and interesting to your friends. Find things to do for those worse off than you are—and one genuinely valuable thing you *can* do is assist in research.

However much scientists accomplish toward the understanding of a baffling disease such as arthritis, they spend little time gloating over these past successes. What is done is dismissed from the mind, once it has been verified as acceptable scientific fact. The things still unknown are what they think about.

It is this kind of intensive search that we call research. To most people, research means working in a laboratory full of gadgets that nobody but the workers themselves could understand. A setup that is not only inexplicable to the average person, but also very expensive, something that could be provided only by a well-stocked endowment fund. This is indeed a valid picture of a research laboratory except that it omits the most important feature of all. In someone's mind an idea was born, an idea which touched off correlative thinking in other minds, to the point where a pattern began to emerge. Excitement builds up. Here is something that must be investigated! Who knows what will be unraveled here—a tangle of useless facts or a discovery that will be a benefit to all mankind? The cold and impartial laboratory results give the answers.

The early career of Albert Einstein gives the best picture I know of the research thinker. Until I read his biography by Ronald W. Clark, my idea of Einstein at work had been in this traditional laboratory setting, surrounded by all the accouterments of physical science and a host of auxiliary workers. This was, in fact, how he earned his living in those early days. But according to his biographer, the work that led him to fame was done after he got home from his job. He would just sit and think, occasionally scribbling a few equations on a scratch pad. One can imagine how this must have looked to his wife, a hardworking woman doing the best she could to give her family a good life on a meager income. She probably knew some women with more cooperative husbands, who lent a hand with household tasks after their own shorter working day had ended. It is not surprising, then, to read that Einstein's first wife left him and took the children to live in Switzerland.

Thinking is the most idle-appearing activity one can indulge in. To the observer, work done inside the skull is truly secret, not much different in appearance from total vacuity. Trying to combine any kind of physical activity, even those mostly directed by the subconscious mind, with this state of concentration becomes extremely hazardous. Well as I thought I knew this, I remember once when I ignored the knowledge to my sorrow. Still bemused by the tribulations of a patient I had just listened to, I pulled out of my parking spot into the path of another car. Fortunately the damage was hardware only, not human.

The reader may well be wondering how all this is concerned with the unsolved problems that still exist in the field of arthritis. Thinking is an involvement we can all share. We can all ask ourselves questions. How could this train of circumstances come about? What else do I know that has a bearing on this patient's symptoms? What are the common points of similarity among the patients I have seen? What other diseases show any hint of relationship to arthritis? Have I dug out all there is of pertinence in this patient's history? How can I be sure that I know what is pertinent and what is not? In all the vast literature now being published about arthritis, are there not leads to solutions of problems now mystifying us that will be plain and clear once they have been pointed out?

If there is any group of people as intimately concerned with the answers to these questions as the health professions are, then it is the group of people who will be reading this book. Most of them will be sufferers from arthritis themselves or suffering from seeing the ravages of the disease upon members of their family. None of these should exclude themselves from the possibility that there may be contributions they can make toward the eradication of the disease. By the time you have finished this book you will know something about the history of arthritis and what theories about it have risen and fallen through the years. You will also know our present views about it, with supporting facts, and the variety of possible explanations that have been offered. Each of you will also have a segment of knowledge peculiar to him or her alone, an individual case history of the disease, perhaps that is exactly like no other that has been written about in the books and journals. Such an individual case history includes not only the facts of the disease, but a knowledge of what it feels like in each stage. In brief, every reader of this book has his own story to tell about arthritis. If one could make a kaleidoscope of all these stories, is it not possible that the reflections might show us things that we have not been able to see otherwise?

193

The major work in any full-scale study of a disease must be done with modern laboratory facilities and trained personnel, but there is always room for ideas from whatever source, and always the possibility that an occasional one of them may strike an illuminating spark of discovery. It seems logical to assume that the more minds there are tuned in to the problems and kept honed to the maximum sheen of receptivity, the more frequently this will occur.

A shining example of the kind of happenstance discovery I am talking about occurred in connection with the recent work on rubella, or German measles. At the time, rubella had about as little attention paid to it as any disease in the medical books, being considered a trivial matter of an infection with a comparatively innocuous virus with very minor morbid possibilities, inflicting no serious damage on any of its victims. Rubella was one sickness a doctor could practically ignore.

The discovery that established rubella as a major cause of a wide variety of birth defects did not come from a pediatrician or an internist, as might be expected. The discovery was made by an Australian ophthalmologist, Dr. Norman Gregg, a kind of doctor who would not even be seeing rubella patients except incidentally, as rubella patients are not apt to have eye complaints of a serious nature.

It was after seeing several cases of cataracts in newborn infants that Dr. Gregg was driven to his fruitful inquiries into the possible causes. He found that the mother of one of these babies had had rubella during her pregnancy. As he found this same thing true of another and then another of his pitiful little patients, he began to suspect that it was something more than coincidence. As he made his suspicions known to others, the path was cleared. Rubella was found to be guilty not only in the matter of cataracts, but as the only virus known to be teratogenetic, or monster-forming.

All this may sound to the reader like a simple matter of deduction on Dr. Gregg's part. Every doctor who sees newborn infants takes a history of the prenatal period, doesn't he? All so true, but not so simple. The kind of routine records a doctor makes on a case may vary a great deal from the kind he makes when he is looking for something specific. It is quite conceivable that several mothers in a row, when questioned about their health during a pregnancy, might forget to mention they had had rubella. If it happened early in the pregnancy, as the most damaging of these attacks do, and they weren't very sick, as they probably were not, it could have faded from their minds almost completely in the six- or seven-month interval before delivery.

Therefore, there was also some cooperative thinking on the part of his patients, which brings us to the next part of the discussion, the part patients may play in solution of their own problems. A good case history is always a necessary adjunct, in fact, to the doctor's best understanding of a case. This has to come from the patient, and the ease and completeness with which it comes can make a great difference in the size of the job the doctor has on his hands.

One thing a patient can always do to help the doctor and economize on the time spent in consultation is to have his history data well in mind before he comes in for his appointment. He can do this best, of course, if he knows what details are significant, what things should be reported. Lacking this knowledge, a patient might spend an hour talking about his illness without coming up with anything pertinent in a strictly medical sense.

I was once feeling very gloomy about the outlook for a patient who had had a stroke. His right side was completely paralyzed, and days had gone by without any sign of improvement. One morning during my routine visit he looked about as usual; he was clear mentally, but rather apathetic. I had looked at the chart, looked at the patient, embarked on a question-and-answer period, without noting any change. My hopes for him were about at an all-time low, when he said, "I forgot to mention. I could move my right foot when I woke up this morning. Does that mean anything?"

It meant everything! He continued to improve, went back to work, and continued in his old job with no apparent physical handicaps.

Patients who have read a book about their particular disease are obviously in a much better position to know what details are medically pertinent. Such a book as this one has attempted to be, is a liaison between the profundity of detail in a medical text and the vocabulary of the general reading public. Which makes the readers of this book eligible as research workers in arthritis. Their work need not be active in a physical sense. People on crutches, in wheelchairs, or bedfast need not be ruled out. All they need is active minds. They all know the basics of arthritis, and each of them knows something else in addition—the individual impact arthritis has had on them. This puts them all in somewhat the same category as that other researcher in arthritis, Thomas Sydenham, whose scientific knowledge about gout was reenforced by his experience in suffering it.

If all the readers of this book ceased to think of

themselves as passive subjects of study and treatment and became active participators in the war against arthritis, who can estimate what progress might be made? The logical place to begin their thinking is in their family backgrounds. Are there hereditary aspects of the disease that have not yet been recognized? I, for one, suspect strongly that there are. Genealogy buffs should be well equipped for such inquiries, and they should widen the scope of their search. They should not stop short at the discovery of some ancestor who was hanged, but try to find out what the rest of them died of. More important still, they should look for information about other concurrent diseases. Gardeners tell me that roots may travel a long way underground and crop up in unexpected places, which suggests an analogical connection with human arthritis.

Not only the names of familial diseases may be important but perhaps the symptomatology also. Look for written records or verbal hand-me-downs of queer things that "seemed to run in the family," even though they were not named accurately—the falling-down fits of Great-Uncle Abner; the several distant cousins that "turned all yellow" in their last years; cases of early senility; family members that got bumps all over their skin; babies that died in their early years of unexplained causes; aunts, great-aunts, and great-great-aunts who developed a jerking sickness that incapacitated them completely before they died; cases of harelip, a backbone that "didn't grow completely closed," "water on the brain" that made the head too big, more than the usual number of fingers and toes, and other developmental anomalies; mongolism and other types of mental retardation.

One may take for granted that the readers of this

book already have in mind cases of arthritis among their relatives and in their immediate family backgrounds. These will have been elicited by their physicians, probably at their first office visit, as a part of the "family history" section of their records. Statements such as "I had several aunts with arthritis," however, are too bare of information. Arthritis is too general, and too varied in its manifestations. Such a statement is little more than a surface indication that there is something worth mining for underneath.

I have found that patients and families of arthritic patients are not apt to refer to the disease by its specific type, such as osteoarthritis or rheumatoid arthritis. When they do, we are that much farther along. When they do not, an attempt should be made to elicit some descriptive information. Important things to note are the age at which the disease appeared, the frequency of remissions, what joints were involved, accessory ailments to which the patient was subject, what treatment the patient had, and the apparent efficacy of it.

The severity of the disease in each subject that is being reported upon should always be noted; whether it was a nagging, discommoding affliction that caused the patient to limp along in his usual line of work, or whether it made of that patient a physical wreck. The dramatic cases, the abject tragedies that have lain for months or years, completely incapacitated, are rather more apt to be handed down in the family records than those whose afflictions have been less torturing. Conscientious researchers, however, will go on digging for nuggets of information among even the mild arthritics, who "weren't really down with it much of the time." In these worst cases, the fixation of multiple joints with the overwhelming catastrophic loss of almost all power of motion, and the loss of mental acuity that may be a concomitant feature, may be a barrier throughout the patient's final months or years to a knowledge of what pathology there may be inside that body. Therefore, there may be even more information to be gleaned from the milder cases.

The family researcher should avoid the pitfall of overlooking possibly important conditions that have existed so long that they have come to be taken for granted by other members of the family. This was the kind of difficulty encountered by the two journalists who collaborated with Jan Welzl in the writing of *Thirty Years in the Golden North*. In the course of his thirty years along the shores of the Arctic in Siberia, Welzl's way of life had become so commonplace to him that he did not volunteer to relate the details. To him, that was "the way things were." Who would want to hear about such everyday things as how the Arctic Ocean sounded when it began to freeze over and masses of ice as large as houses were broken up by the tides and hurled onto the shore? It was true, he admitted, that some men went crazy from the terror of it. But since it happened every year, it was not unique to him. It was only by persistent digging and prodding that his interrogaters elicited a full-scale description from him.

To be as objective as possible in reporting these family ills should be the aim of the researcher. It means the sometimes difficult task of asking oneself, "How would this look to me if I were an outsider, not a member of the family but someone who has come upon the case as an onlooker?" Some intimately involved relatives might even find it impossible to take such a position. For them, a collaboration with several others might solve the difficulty, thus obtaining a multifaceted image.

With this multiplicity of selection of subjects for a multitude of interested people to think and wonder about, is it not likely that discoveries of importance should be forthcoming?

The amateur researcher in arthritis is apt to come to his job all fired up, goggle-eyed, and trusting. Everything seems new and interesting to him. How could it help being important? "I talked to twelve arthritics today, and all but two of them had high blood pressure too. Doesn't that mean there must be a connection?"

Now he learns for the first time the difference between significance and coincidence. Arthritis is such a common disease that coincidence is the most frequent blight on its research. Any disease in the textbook could be hooked up with arthritis without making an event worthy of notice. In fact, the opposite situation, a paucity of arthritis, has been considered of sufficient significance to deserve comment. (This was the study that showed the inmates of penal institutions to be freer of arthritis than the general populace.)

The determined researcher, however, will not allow himself to be buffaloed by coincidence. If he knows a case of arthritis associated with a comparatively rare disease, even that one case may be worth reporting. He has to start somewhere, doesn't he? So he should throw it out on the table, face up, and see if any of the other players can match it. If one or more of them can, he may be in business. He may be on the trail of some important discovery.

To start the game going, I'll throw out one such single-instance case of mine. One of the most severe cases of ankylosing spondylitis I ever saw was the son of a woman with multiple sclerosis. Does that mean anything? I have often wondered, but have found nothing in the literature with any bearing on it.

This one-case reporting must not get out of hand, however, or we should only complicate things. To be eligible for attention, such a case must have had some continued impact on the mind, some persistent needling effect that does not permit its being cast aside and forgotten.

It seems to me that one of the most promising sources of new knowledge should be the juvenile type of rheumatoid arthritis. Any obscure disease that strikes a patient sometime in infancy automatically raises the possibility of familial factors. Continuing search for hereditary sidelights should be in order here. This childhood form of the disease is much rarer than the adult form, and therefore it should be possible to give more research attention to individual cases. Any new fact uncovered is likely to have a bearing on the whole rheumatoid family, as the connection between the juvenile and adult types seems indisputable. Who knows but that some of the missing pieces of the puzzle might lie in the backgrounds of these afflicted children?

Anything that grows may undergo mutations from one generation to the next, changes originating in the genes or chromosomes in response to stimuli, or as adaptations to environmental necessities. Thus the same disease may present various aspects in different subjects, or at different stages of observation. The predominating finding in one patient may be entirely lacking in another. Ills of a previous generation may stamp a child with a morbid sign quite unlike what

201

shows in the parent. For example, mothers who have had German measles during pregnancy often give birth to babies who have cataracts in their eyes.

A patient struck by a disease before the age of two does not have a very long personal history, but the roots of his family history go back for generations. Many of them are perhaps hidden forever, but as many of them as possible should be brought to light.

I have mentioned the needling effect that some cases have on the observer. The case of juvenile rheumatoid arthritis that has needled me into all this discourse is one in which there is a family background of Huntington's chorea. The persistence of Huntington's chorea in successive generations is well known, enough to make it suspect in any of the other ills of the family. I have found nothing in the literature about any connection between it and arthritis. So here is another card I lay on the table, face up. Are there any matches?

Index

years of this disease appear other than passive, resigned, long-suffering?

So many personality traits have been reported as
"typical" of the premorbid arthritic temperament that
if one tried to avoid arthritis by subduing all of them,
he would have to cancel out his personality altogether
and become a robot. I do not wish to impugn the validity of any of these studies or to intimate that they are
without value. Their value increases as they are repeated by other groups in other places, under varying
circumstances. The inevitable results of such labors will
be to sift out the nuggets of truth.

Among the adjectives that have been claimed to
describe the arthritic personality are shy, rigid, moralis-
tic, inhibited, self-conscious, conforming, self-sacrific-
ing, masochistic, perfectionistic. Schizophrenic is on
the list of some observers, who claim to have found
similarities between rheumatoid arthritics and schiz-
ophrenics. If these observers are correct, the fact that
it is most unusual for the two diseases to occur in the
same person would suggest that some of these individuals eventually come to a point at which, however unwit-
tingly, they make a choice between arthritis and schizophrenia.

There must be some connection or some kind of
relationship, between what we call rheumatoid arthritis and what we call schizophrenia, because of the
demonstrated fact that the incidence of arthritis in hospitalized psychotics, who are preponderantly schizo-
phrenics, is significantly less than in the population as
a whole. Dr. D. Gregg published a paper in the *American Journal of Psychiatry* on the paucity of arthritis
among psychotic cases, in which he states that only

103

twenty cases of arthritis were reported in more than fifteen thousand hospitalized psychotics. Allusion has been made in previous chapters to the poorly defined boundaries of rheumatoid arthritis. Trying to correlate this disease with schizophrenia (which psychiatrist R. D. Laing says has no definition at all and may not even exist as an entity) seems a more erratic journey into uncharted space than a discussion which is trying to remain rooted on solid scientific ground.

Any kind of scientist feels himself out on a limb, naked to the scorn of exacting colleagues, unless he can clothe his beliefs in some kind of explanatory garment, however flimsy. So we listen willingly to any theories that sound logical.

One of these has to do with the body's natural immune protective mechanisms, which have a well-proven status. Normally the body has the power to throw out defenses, even attacking forces, against a great many ills that threaten it. Among these are the armies of white cells produced to combat infection; antibodies against specific diseases; injection of extra adrenaline into the blood stream to speed up reaction in time of danger. It seems logical to assume that there are many more that we do not know about. A suggestion of the theorists is that when everything in the body is in normal working order, something, probably one of the endocrine glands, issues an internal prescription for some kind of protective balm to the joints. When anything disrupts the communication system, the order does not get through, and the joints are left vulnerable.

This disrupting factor may well be an emotional one—grief, anger, anxiety, worry, disappointment, discouragement, depression. While these emotions are the common lot of us all, history shows that the damaging